Intermittent Fasting For Women Over 50

Complete Guide to Lose Weight, Restore Metabolism, Promote Longevity, Increase Energy, and Detox the Body in a Healthy and Simple Way

Phyliss Andie Kayleen

© Copyright 2021 - All rights reserved.

The content contained within this book may not be reproduced, duplicated, or transmitted without direct written permission from the author or the publisher.

Under no circumstances will any blame or legal responsibility be held against the publisher, or author, for any damages, reparation, or monetary loss due to the information contained within this book, either directly or indirectly.

Legal Notice:

This book is copyright protected. It is only for personal use. You cannot amend, distribute, sell, use, quote, or paraphrase any part, or the content within this book, without the consent of the author or publisher.

Disclaimer Notice:

Please note the information contained within this document is for educational and entertainment purposes only. All effort has been executed to present accurate, up-to-date, reliable, complete information. No warranties of any kind are declared or implied. Readers acknowledge that the author is not engaged in the rendering of legal, financial, medical, or professional advice. The content within this book has been derived from various sources. Please consult a licensed professional before attempting any techniques outlined in this book.

By reading this document, the reader agrees that under no circumstances is the author responsible for any losses, direct or indirect, that are incurred as a result of the use of the information contained within this document, including, but not limited to, errors, omissions, or inaccuracies.

Table of Contents

Introduction 9

Chapter 1: What Is Intermittent Fasting? 11

    How Intermittent Fasting Works 14

        Combining Intermittent Fasting and the Ketogenic Diet 15

        How to Incorporate Keto Into Your Intermittent Fasting Plan 15

    Choosing Your Intervals 18

        The Eight Hour Eating Interval or 16:8 18

        The 5:2 Approach 19

        The 36-Hour Protocol 19

        The 42-Hour Protocol 20

        The Eat Stop Eat Protocol 20

        The Warrior Fast 20

    The Benefits of Intermittent Fasting 21

Chapter 2: Shopping List 23

Chapter 3: Keto Breakfast Recipes 24

    Bacon, Egg, & Cheese Breakfast Muffins 25

    Blueberry Almond Pancakes 27

    Berry Breakfast Shake 29

    Cheddar, Spinach, & Mushroom Omelet 30

    Delicious Poached Eggs 32

    Frittata With Feta and Green Onion 34

    Red and Green Frittata 36

Spicey, Bacon Omelet 38

Bacon and Cheese Ham Steaks 40

Cheesy French Style Omelet 42

Savory Sausage and Sage Patties 44

Popeye's Mushroom Scramble 46

Triple Threat Quiche Cups 48

Cheesy-Greens Mediterranean Omelet 50

Smooth and Creamy Asparagus Omelet 52

Keto-Friendly Spinach Quiche 54

Greens, Eggs, and Ham 56

Mile High Omelet 58

Tri-Color Scramble 60

Avo Bacon Scramble 62

Rustic Apple-Turkey Sausage Patties 64

Swiss Cheese "Zittata" 66

Two-Bite Breakfast Bakes 68

Frittata Italiana 70

The Cheesy Classic 72

Rainbow Frittata 74

Bacon Wrapped Egg Bites 76

Chapter 4: Keto Lunch Recipes 78

Simple Cauli-Floret Mac 'n Cheese 79

Keto Beef Egg Roll in a Bowl 81

Cobb Salad 83

Classic Shrimp Scampi with Keto Broccoli 'Noodles' 85

Portobello Pizza Pies 87

Easy Cheesy Keto Beef Bowls 89

Pescatarian Surf 'N' Turf 91

Keto-Friendly Tuna Salad.. 93

Winter's Afternoon Spaghetti Squash 94

Not-So-Starchy Risotto 96

Sweet and Savory Chicken Lettuce Wraps 98

Korean Beef and Rice for Keto 100

Fast-Breaking Chili..102

Avocados Con Taco..104

Buffalo Shrimp Lettuce Wraps 106

Broccoli Salad for Keto 108

Keto-Friendly Egg Salad.. 110

Bacon Sushi Rolls 112

Fat Bomb Burger Bites 114

Winter Asian Beef Salad With a Twist 116

Pizza Fatta Con Zucchini 118

Garlic and Herb Roasted Chicken Thighs.............120

Chicken Niçoise Salad 122

Finger Licking Grilled Turkey With Dill 124

Shakshuka..126

Chapter 5: Keto Dinner Recipes 128

Kimchi Pork Lettuce Cups....................................129

Thai Turkey Burgers 131

BBQ Flank Steak & Cabbage Slaw........................133

Zoodle Beef Bolognese..135

Smoky Butter Roasted Chicken 137

Chicken Fajita Bowls... 139

Almond-Crusted Salmon Patties 142

Swedish Meatballs.. 144

Magic Keto Pizza 146

Salmon Wrapped in a Parcel... 148

Low Calorie Broiled Chicken With Parmesan Artichokes
.... 150

Melt in Your Mouth Steak..152

Zoodles with Herby Tilapia...154

Smoky Scallops and Spinach 156

Thai Cauliflower Soup... 158

Punchy Dill Chicken... 160

Steak and Eggs With a Warm Summer Salad 162

Spicy Mexican Cabbage and Green Chili Soup............ 164

Classic BLT With a Twist 166

Grecian Ribeye Steaks... 168

Chapter 6: Keto Snack Recipes 170

Smoky Cheese Dip... 171

Italian Antipasto Cheese Ring 173

French Tapenade With Red Peppers and Almonds 175

Chicken-Cheese Skewers 177

Pimiento and Cheese Deviled Eggs...................................179

Smoky Salmon Cream Cheese Dip....................................181

Sweet Red Pepper Seasoned Cheese............................... 183

Italian Style Portobello Mushrooms............................... 185

Summer Fresh Chicken Dip...187

Cheese and Chives Ball 189

Creamy Parmesan Caulimash 191

Sausage Stuffed Mushrooms Caps 193

Cream Cheese and Pork Stuffed Jalapenos 195

Asparagus in a Blanket 197

Garlic and Parmesan Spinach Bake 199

Pigs in a Jalapeno Blanket... 201

Piacenza Asparagus 203

Cheesy Portobello Mushrooms..................................... 205

Roquefort Jumbo Shrimp.. 207

Spicy Pecan Cheese Spread 209

Italian-Style Artichoke Hearts....................................... 211

Texan Poppers with Spicy Sausage Dip........................ 213

Zesty Broccoli Roast 215

Spinach and Cheese Marinara Dip............................... 217

Black and White Truffles 219

Waist-Friendly Chocolate Cups.................................... 221

Cheddar Cheese Crisps 223

Bumblebee Muffins 224

Keto Butter Cookies.. 226

Cheesy Breakfast Biscuits... 228

Parmesan Zucchini Fries 230

Chapter 7: Meal Plan and Exercise Plan............................ 232

Week 1.. 232

Week 2 233

Week 3 234

Week 4 236
Exercise Plan 238
   Strength Training for Over 240
   Yoga For Over 50s 241
   Cardio for Over 50s 243
   1 Week Workout Schedule 244
Conclusion 246
References 250

Introduction

Studied in laboratories and used throughout the world, intermittent fasting (IF) is fast becoming an international phenomenon. IF is not a fad but a healthy, beneficial way to lose weight, reduce low-density lipoprotein (LDL)–also known as 'bad cholesterol'– and improve overall heart and body health. It has significant positive effects on many aspects of people's lives by following the body's natural circadian rhythms when it comes to eating. As the trend of intermittent fasting spread throughout the world, more focus was placed on the benefits of this natural way of eating for individuals over the age of 50.

Weight loss and maintaining a healthy balance within the body can be challenging for women over age 50 as they often have unique, and sometimes complex, health issues. Severely restrictive diets or fad trends that encourage starvation may have moderately negative effects on women in their younger years but, after age 50, these approaches can be devastating to a woman's health. The risks of osteoporosis, osteoarthritis, menopausal hormone deficiencies, heart disease, and high blood pressure all significantly increase after the age of 50. When severely restrictive diets are implemented, health risks increase and the consequences can be irreversible.

Intermittent fasting does not promote starvation or severely restricting calorie intake. Instead, it seeks to create a natural balance with the body's circadian rhythm (or wake and sleep cycle) to ensure that you are getting the right nutrition at the right time. In a fast-paced world that focuses on convenience, eating unhealthy processed foods is common. These foods, which are high in salt and chemical preservatives, throw the body into an unhealthy cycle–one that can drive obesity. If a lack of exercise and high stress levels are also factors, these unhealthy habits may seem impossible to break.

Because intermittent fasting works with the body's natural cycles, poor habits–related to both eating and exercise–become easier to eliminate. Recent Harvard studies have shown that IF in both animals and people flips the mitochondria in the body, encouraging them to work more efficiently, doing their specific jobs at night instead of assisting in the digestive processes (Tello, 2020). What is vital to remember is that intermittent fasting is only effective if done correctly. This means that your required caloric intake should be met but only during the hours outside of your fasting period. This flips the metabolic switch in your body, triggering all of the right digestive and fuel creation responses.

Many would argue that it is difficult to find a downside to intermittent fasting.

Now that you know the benefits of intermittent fasting, can you afford not to incorporate healthy intermittent fasting into your life?

Chapter 1: What Is Intermittent Fasting?

Intermittent fasting is fast becoming one of the world's most popular health and fitness trends but is often misunderstood. Many believe that it involves being hungry for extended periods. I would like to make it clear from the outset that intermittent fasting does not encourage a person to starve themselves.

Because the dietary requirements of IF are less restrictive than that of other eating plans, more and more people are showing interest in this age-old way of eating. Intermittent fasting does not fixate so much on the exact makeup of the diet. Rather, it focuses on the time and time between meals when a person should eat to lose weight, build muscle, or healthily maintain their weight. This means that a person will follow their usual healthy calorie allowance, but will only permit themselves to eat in their allotted eating timeframe.

Whether or not you are actively practicing intermittent fasting, when you sleep at night, your body is in a fasting state. During your nightly rest period of (ideally) six to eight hours your body fasts, unless you wake during the night to eat. This period of non-eating is called a "fasting window." If you do not snack in the middle of the night, your first meal of the day breaks your fast which is why your morning meal is called 'breakfast.' When you eat during the day, your body enters a 'fed state' which encourages the digestive process to absorb food converting it to energy.

Eating plans that dictate what a person can and cannot eat can be difficult to maintain. They are often costly and involve weighing food or counting macronutrients. For some, the cost and effort required to maintain the recommended way of eating are not worth the undue stress. In addition, the restrictive nature of most of these eating plans can create unwanted health issues and drive cravings, as whole food groups are left out. Intermittent fasting, on the other hand, encourages the consumer to eat to satiation within their prescribed daily calorie allowance.

When you embark on your intermittent fasting journey, it is important to remember that fasting has less to do with 'what' you should be eating and more to do with 'when' you should be eating. With time, your body will get used to the intervals of fasting and eating and your appetite will slowly decrease. Cravings, particularly for sugar, may occur as your body initially adjusts but these will subside over time. Intermittent fasting requires far less self-discipline than restrictive eating plans. This is because the individual is permitted to eat the way they are accustomed to while still being mindful of how many calories they are consuming.

Intermittent fasting requires you to question the reasons why you feel the need to eat. Before embarking on your IF journey ask yourself a few critical questions.

Do I often find myself eating at odd hours of the day?

Am I an emotional eater?

Do I find myself reaching for unhealthy snacks, even in the middle of the night?

Are there specific times of the day when I feel my energy crashing?

What do I crave during these low-energy moments?

How much of my diet is made up of artificial sugars and processed foods?

Do I get up during the night to eat?

The answers to these questions will give you a better idea of why you are craving unhealthy foods and will also help you to gain a better understanding of when your fasting window should be. For most people, an energy slump occurs around midday. This is because they fuel their body with the wrong foods, or no food, in the morning. The body depletes its energy resources too quickly and sugar cravings usually occur (Duan et al., 2016).

To better understand how our digestive system and metabolic action works, you need to understand the role of insulin in your body. Insulin determines what happens to the food you eat. It dictates what is turned into energy and what is stored as fat. If you eat excessively and live a sedentary lifestyle, most of the food you consume will be turned into fat. Much of the processed, high-fat, sugary foods available to us spike insulin levels. This means that, while you may not be full after eating a fast-food burger on the run, your body is producing high levels of insulin and converting that food to fat rather than sustainable energy (Carter, 2019). Regular consumption of processed foods will create high levels of insulin that remain in your body for unhealthy and extended periods. This elevated level of insulin over an extended period creates insulin resistance, a condition whereby your body can no longer effectively process fat into energy (Divers, 2020). For the body to maintain or lose weight, it requires consistent, longer periods of low insulin. Intermittent fasting encourages these lowered insulin periods by promoting sustained periods of non-eating. It is important to understand that even healthy foods cause moderate spikes in your insulin levels but the spikes are less extreme and are more easily regulated by the body (Carter, 2019).

How Intermittent Fasting Works

Intermittent fasting is defined by periods of non-eating. The difference between intermittent fasting and your natural evening fast is the lengthening of your fasting window. For example, you may follow a fasting program that requires you to fast for 16 hours and eat your meals during an 8-hour window. In this case, if your first meal is at 8:00 a.m., your last meal should be at 4:00 p.m. This 16-hour by 8-hour program is called a 'fasting protocol.'

During your 16-hour fasting window, you can consume liquids like water, black unsweetened tea, and black unsweetened coffee as these are considered to be 'zero calorie' fluids. While I have used the 16/8 protocol as an example, it is not the only way to fast. Shifting your fasting plan, or choosing a protocol that fits within your lifestyle, will make it easier to follow.

During your fasting window, your body will undergo a metabolic switch and change its source of energy; this means your body will start to use your fat reserves for energy. In essence, fat is converted into ketones so that the body can sustain its energy levels.

In the initial phases of intermittent fasting, you may have some feelings of hunger, but those feelings are rarely because your body requires food to fuel itself. Rather, these feelings of hunger are cravings for sugar to spike insulin levels in the way your body has become accustomed. These cravings and feelings of hunger will dissipate quite quickly as your body begins to draw on its energy reserves when needed.

Combining Intermittent Fasting and the Ketogenic Diet

The connection between intermittent fasting and a ketogenic diet is ketosis. Ketosis is the metabolic switch that occurs within the body when stored fats are converted to energy. When this fat is broken down, ketones are produced. These ketone molecules are used to sustain energy levels (during periods when the person is not eating. While intermittent fasting can work on a carb-centric diet, it is most effective when combined with a keto diet because it speeds up the ketosis process. The ketogenic diet reduces complex carbohydrates from your diet to keep the body in a sustained ketosis state. When used in conjunction with IF, this sustained state of ketosis will reduce body fat quickly without affecting lean muscle mass. Combining intermittent fasting with a ketogenic diet plan is particularly useful in overcoming weight loss plateaus (Migala, 2019) and can be incredibly effective in regulating diabetes-related insulin issues.

How to Incorporate Keto Into Your Intermittent Fasting Plan

It is important to ease yourself into incorporating both keto and intermittent fasting into your dietary routines. I recommend that you first introduce your body to a ketogenic diet and give yourself time to adjust to the new flavors, as well as fewer complex carbohydrates. For the first two weeks, eat a keto-friendly diet, slowly substituting healthier alternatives for complex carbohydrates. During this keto adjustment period take note of when you are genuinely hungry and focus on learning to differentiate between hunger and sugar cravings.

Once you have become accustomed to your new diet, you can begin fasting. Ideally, your last meal of the day should be eaten no later than 7 p.m. However, adjustments may be needed for you to fast for the required number of hours. For shift workers and those who work at night, the time of the final meal of the day will need to be adjusted.

The 16/8 (or eight-hour) eating interval is the most common method but it is important to choose a protocol that suits your lifestyle. I have included descriptions of the most popular IF protocols.

Once your eating interval has been established, set your health or weight loss goals, determine what your ideals for your body are, as well as the reasons why you want to change your eating patterns. These reasons could include wanting to lose weight, gain muscle, live a healthier lifestyle, etc. Be clear and concise in your reasons for wanting to change so you remain motivated to achieve results. Once you have determined the reason(s) you want to make changes, you will need to ascertain what your caloric needs are for your specific objectives. This is because the purpose—why you are fasting (weight maintenance, muscle gain, or weight loss) have different caloric requirements. Knowing the number of calories you need to consume in a day will assist you in breaking down your nutritional requirements per meal, helping ensure that you never feel excessively hungry.

This book does contain a sample eating plan but feel free to mix and match the recipes to suit your specific needs and tastes. Make sure to plan your meals in advance to avoid slipping into bad habits or substituting quick-to-grab unhealthy snacks for healthy food choices.

Meal planning is not only beneficial to your budget but for keeping your health goals on track. You will need to keep in mind that not all calories are created equal. Foods that are nutritionally dense and high in protein provide great nutrition while preventing feelings of hunger.

Finally, with all of your proactive steps in place, you will need to plan how, when, and which of the suggested protocols you will use. Once you begin your fasting plan, make sure that you revisit, not only your goals but the reasons why you are on your intermittent fasting and keto journey.

Stay motivated and celebrate all of your weight, strength, health, and fitness accomplishments so that your new lifestyle remains one that is rewarding to you.

Choosing Your Intervals

The list of options for your intermittent fasting program is, thankfully, not extensive. There are no hard and fast rules when it comes to choosing a fasting protocol. Each interval has advantages and disadvantages. Protocols can be mixed and matched, should you wish. If you want to incorporate more exercise into your regime, the eight-hour interval may be the best option for you. If you wish to lose weight quickly, but healthily, the 5:2 approach may suit your needs.

Intermittent fasting works well using all protocols, but some are not meant to be sustained for long periods. It is vitally important to do your research so you can find a fasting routine that works for you.

The Eight Hour Eating Interval or 16:8

To institute the 16:8 protocol, you eat only during an eight-hour window of the day and fast for the remainder. For example, you may choose to eat between the hours of 11 a.m. and 7 p.m. As previously mentioned, it is better to coordinate your fasting window with your sleep patterns. If you were to set 11 a.m. to 7 p.m. as your eating period, as mentioned previously, your fasting period would be 7 p.m. to 10 a.m. The fact that you are sleeping during a portion of that time means you will be naturally fasting during those hours; the amount of time that you will have to abstain from eating is decreased when your fasting period and sleep time overlap.

When merging fasting and sleeping, you are following your body's natural circadian rhythm. This will make it easier to deal with feelings of hunger or unhealthy snack habits. Upon waking, do some light stretching or an aerobic exercise routine for 10 minutes, then eat a satiating meal like our Mile High Omelet (recipe included in a later section) to replenish your energy for the remainder of the day. Lunch can be eaten around midday. Depending on how long you are awake, and your caloric requirements, a small amount can be eaten after 3 p.m.; do not eat after 6 p.m. The idea is that you do not eat for 16 consecutive hours of your day.

The 5:2 Approach

The 5:2 approach requires you to eat your normal calorie intake for five days and restrict your caloric intake to 500 calories on the remaining two days. To implement the 5:2 approach, eat your usual calorie intake on Monday, Wednesday, Thursday, Saturday, and Sunday, restricting your calories on Tuesday and Friday. Most find this method to be extremely effective for losing weight quickly, but it should not be used continuously. The reason for this is, eventually, the body may perceive itself to be starving and will begin to slow its metabolism.

The 36-Hour Protocol

36-hour fasting protocols require you to fast for an entire day. For example, on day one you would eat normally (with your last meal being eaten at 7 p.m.). Day two would require you to skip all meals for 24 hours meaning you would not eat again until breakfast on the morning of day three.

Some dieticians recommend the 36-hour protocol to assist in stabilizing insulin levels in sufferers of type 2 diabetes.

The 42-Hour Protocol

As described above, when using the 36-hour protocol, you break your fast on the morning of day three. When using the 42-hour protocol, you continue fasting until noon on day three.

When instituting longer fasting periods, you should not consider calorie intake; you should eat to satiation rather than counting your calories when breaking your fast.

Once again, dieticians sometimes recommend this protocol for those who have type 2 diabetes who are insulin resistant. Many people can maintain this schedule for one or two weeks. It is not recommended that this protocol be used often or for extended periods.

The Eat Stop Eat Protocol

This protocol involves fasting for a full 24 hours, twice a week. This method was popularized by fitness experts who recommended refraining from eating for a full 24 hours after an evening meal to promote fat burning.

An easy way to institute the eat stop eat method is as follows: Monday, Wednesday, Thursday, Saturday, and Sunday, eat according to the 16/8 approach, fasting a full 24 hours on Tuesday and Friday. During your 24-hour fasting period, water, tea, coffee, as well as other calorie-free beverages are permitted but no foods or drinks that contain calories are allowed.

The Warrior Fast

The warrior fast works well with a ketogenic diet for people looking to lose weight consistently. Popular among nutritionists, warrior fasting involves loosely fasting by snacking lightly during daylight hours and eating to satiation at supper time. A typical warrior fast involves vegetables from an approved list, that can be eaten all day, and a large main meal comprising the remainder of your keto calories in the evening.

The Benefits of Intermittent Fasting

Aside from the obvious benefit of healthy weight loss, intermittent fasting comes with a host of other benefits. Within the first few days of beginning your fasting program, glucose levels begin to balance out, helping to fuel your body more efficiently. LDL cholesterol levels begin to drop during the first month of fasting. This balances high-density lipoprotein (HDL), 'good cholesterol,' in your body. The lowering of LDL cholesterol improves liver function and heart health.

Eating according to your circadian rhythm, which means no food after sundown, promotes good, uninterrupted deep sleep. New research indicates that intermittent fasting may be linked to decreases in the growth of cancerous tumors, specifically those associated with breast cancer (Huizen, 2021).

As women age, hormones and less active lifestyles tend to result in extra weight in the midsection. As you know, weight loss is a major benefit of intermittent fasting, but did you know that IF targets stubborn belly fat? A 2014 scientific review on intermittent fasting showed that, not only did the participants of the study drop an average of 5% of their body weight per week but that a person's waist circumference was most affected by this weight loss (Welton et al, 2020). The Harvard Medical School states that belly fat is particularly dangerous in women as it increases the risk of heart disease and heart attacks by 18% (Bilodeau, 2018). Intermittent fasting helps reduce the risk of heart disease by eradicating belly fat as well as hormonal hip fat deposits. These fat deposits are formed as a result of increased levels of estrogen and progesterone, a hormone that is prevalent in women (Bird, 2002).

Additional studies have shown that fasting reduces oxidative stress, a process that causes inflammation in the body. Intermittent fasting increases the body's ability to respond to this oxidative process, alleviating the symptoms of arthritis, psoriasis, and chronic joint inflammation.

Finally, IF has been shown to promote healing on a cellular level, through initiating the waste disposal response within the body's mitochondria. The body's cells, instead of processing late-night foods and snacks, return to their natural function of removing toxins from the body. This function greatly reduces the risk of certain cancers, Alzheimer's disease, and other degenerative diseases.

Chapter 2: Shopping List

Fermented foods: pickles, kimchi, sauerkraut, plain full-fat yogurt.

Nuts and seeds: almonds, walnuts, macadamia nuts, brazil nuts, pecans, chia seeds, pumpkin seeds, sunflower seeds, sesame seeds, almond flour, or meal, coconut flour.

Oils: avocado oil, extra virgin olive oil, cold-pressed or virgin coconut oil, ghee, MCT oil

Spices and sweeteners: red pepper flakes, basil, oregano, bay leaves, smoked paprika, sea salts, black pepper, cumin, curry powder, 'everything' bagel seasoning, whole-grain mustard, stevia, monk fruit sweetener.

Canned goods and other shelf-stable items: coconut cream, coconut milk, almond milk, olives, dark chocolate, cocoa powder, tea and coffee, pork rinds, baking powder.

Perishables: bacon and sausage, eggs, coconut wraps, low-carb tortillas, sugar-free mayonnaise, heavy cream, low-carb bread or rolls, butter, cheese, Parmesan.

Chapter 3: Keto Breakfast Recipes

For anyone living with chronic illness, including type 2 diabetes, or who has difficulty processing sugars, the importance of eating a low carbohydrate diet is well known. When on an intermittent fasting plan you need to institute balanced nutritious meals that fuel your body. By fueling your body the right way, you can maintain your energy levels throughout the day. For those who do not eat a well-balanced breakfast, the largest blood sugar spike of the day comes with their first meal. This is because non-keto fasters usually grab quick, but unhealthy meals, on their way to work. Sugary cereals, toast with jam, fruits, and refined oats–not to mention drive-through takeaway meals–send sugar levels skyrocketing.

Consuming a low carbohydrate breakfast that provides your body with adequate nutrition, prevents blood sugar spikes and the associated symptoms. Pre-lunch hunger, as well as the urge to eat sugary snacks, begins to diminish as the body becomes accustomed to a healthy meal to start the day. This is because a low-carb breakfast reduces your energy intake as your body metabolizes the nutrients throughout the day.

Preliminary studies on type 2 diabetics have shown the true power of eating a keto breakfast in the morning with more than 50% of diabetics showing signs of their disease going into remission when eating a ketogenic diet while instituting intermittent fasting (Marengo, 2020).

Bacon, Egg, & Cheese Breakfast Muffins

An easy, filling meal, these bacon, egg, and cheese muffins can be prepared the night before and grabbed in the morning, for an on-the-go meal as you get on with your day.

Time: 40 minutes

Serving Size: 6 servings

Prep Time: 10 minutes

Cook Time: 30 minutes

Nutritional Facts/Info:

Calories 303

Carbs 1.5 g

Fat 26 g

Protein 15 g

Ingredients:

- 6 slices bacon
- 8 eggs
- ¼ cup heavy cream
- Fine sea salt and freshly ground black pepper to taste
- 3 ounces shredded cheddar cheese

Directions:

1. Preheat your oven to 375 degrees.
2. Generously grease a 6-cup muffin tin with butter.
3. Using a skillet, cook bacon over medium-high heat. (The length of time required to fry the bacon depends on

personal preference.) Place the bacon on a paper towel-lined plate to drain the excess grease.
4. Cut or crumble the bacon.
5. In a deep bowl, whisk the eggs, cream, salt, and pepper. Make sure that everything is well combined.
6. Add bacon pieces and some cheese, sprinkling an even amount of both into each cup of the muffin tin.
7. Pour the egg mixture equally into the muffin cups.
8. Bake for 20 to 25 minutes, or until the eggs puff up and are slightly golden.
9. Serve and enjoy!

Blueberry Almond Pancakes

Who doesn't love the smell of fresh pancakes in the morning? Low in calories and carbohydrates, our blueberry almond pancakes can be made in double batches and frozen for later.

Time: 10 minutes

Serving Size: 10 pancakes

Prep Time: 5 minutes

Cook Time: 5 minutes

Nutritional Facts/Info:

Calories 114

Carbs 3.9 g

Fat 10 g

Protein 3.9 g

Ingredients:

- 4 tablespoons butter
- ¼ cup almond milk
- 2 large eggs
- ¾ cup almond flour
- ¼ teaspoon pure vanilla extract
- 1 teaspoon baking powder
- 1 tablespoon flax meal
- ¼ teaspoon sea salt
- 1 packet stevia powder
- ¾ cup blueberries, frozen
- ¼ tsp allspice (optional)
- Fresh butter, to cook the pancakes

Directions:

1. Using a whisk, in a small bowl, combine the butter, almond milk, vanilla, and eggs. Make sure that everything is well combined.
2. To your wet ingredients, add the flax meal, flour, baking powder, stevia, salt, and allspice. Mix until well combined.
3. Add the blueberries.
4. Heat a nonstick skillet over medium heat. (When you think your skillet is well-heated, try adding a few drops of water. If the drops dance across the surface, your skillet is at optimal temperature.)
5. Add butter to the skillet. Spread so there is a thin layer over the entire skillet.
6. Scoop ¼ cup of batter into the skillet, spreading it out into a thin circle.
7. Cook for 1 to 2 minutes, or until bubbles appear and pop and the edges begin to form.
8. Flip and cook for another 1 to 2 minutes.
9. Serve hot and enjoy!

Berry Breakfast Shake

Perfect for the person who prefers a lighter breakfast, this berry breakfast shake is easy to make and is packed with vitamins and minerals.

Time: 5 minutes

Serving Size: 1 serving

Prep Time: 5 minutes

Cook Time: 0 minutes

Nutritional Facts/Info:

Calories 900

Carbs 18 g

Fat 80 g

Protein 10 g

Ingredients:

- ¼ cup frozen mixed berries
- ½ cup coconut or almond milk
- ½ cup heavy cream
- ½ tsp fresh squeezed lemon juice
- 1 tbsp almond butter
- 1 tbsp MCT oil (optional)

Directions:

1. Add all the ingredients to your blender jug.
2. Blend until smooth.
3. Serve immediately and enjoy.

Cheddar, Spinach, & Mushroom Omelet

A hearty fall or winter meal, this omelet fills the gap for anyone who wakes up hungry. Also perfect for a post-workout meal to boost muscle-building proteins.

Time: 10 minutes

Serving Size: 2 servings

Prep Time: 4 minutes

Cook Time: 6 minutes

Nutritional Facts/Info:

Calories 500

Carbs 5 g

Fat 38 g

Protein 34 g

Ingredients:

- 2 teaspoons extra virgin olive oil
- 2 cups packed baby spinach
- sea salt to taste
- a handful of fresh parsley, chopped
- 3 ounces white button mushrooms, sliced
- 4 ounces cheddar cheese, shredded
- 6 large eggs, lightly beaten

Directions:

1. Using an 8-inch nonstick skillet, heat 1 teaspoon of oil over medium-high heat until the oil glistens or shimmers.
2. Add the mushrooms and cook for 3 to 4 minutes, stirring occasionally, until the mushrooms are golden brown on all sides.
3. Add the spinach and season with salt.
4. Cook the spinach until it wilts (about 1 to 2 minutes).
5. Transfer the spinach and mushroom mixture to a bowl. Stir in the parsley and set aside.
6. In a separate bowl, lightly beat 6 large eggs and season with salt.
7. Heat the remaining teaspoon of oil in the same skillet. Pour the eggs into the pan, swirling the mixture until the eggs are evenly distributed across the bottom of the pan.
8. Cook without disturbing the eggs until the edges are set.
9. Using a rubber spatula, lift the edges of the egg, while tilting the pan. This will allow any uncooked egg to slide down to the cooking surface of the pan and cook.
10. Once cooked evenly, cover one-half of the eggs with the vegetable mixture. Top with cheese.
11. Fold the plain portion of the omelet over the spinach and mushroom portion, creating a half-moon, and cook for an additional minute.
12. Serve immediately and enjoy.

Delicious Poached Eggs

Classy and traditional, keto poached eggs are the perfect Sunday brunch after a long fast.

Time: 45 minutes

Serving Size: 4 servings

Prep Time: 10 minutes

Cook Time: 35 minutes

Nutritional Facts/Info:

Calories 300

Carbs 22 g

Fat 12 g

Protein 14 g

Ingredients:

- 3 garlic cloves, minced
- 1 white onion, chopped
- 1 tablespoon ghee
- Salt and black pepper to taste
- 1 serrano pepper, chopped
- 3 tomatoes, chopped
- 1 red bell pepper, chopped
- 1 tsp cumin
- 1 tsp paprika
- 1 tbsp cilantro, chopped
- ¼ teaspoon chili powder
- 6 eggs

Directions:

1. Add ghee to the pan and heat over medium heat.
2. Add onions and cook until soft (approximately 10 minutes).
3. Add the serrano pepper and garlic. Stir and cook for 1 minute.
4. Add the red bell pepper. Stir and cook for another 10 minutes.
5. Add tomatoes, salt, pepper, chili powder, cumin, and paprika, stir and cook for 10 minutes. Make sure to stir well to combine all the flavors.
6. Crack eggs into the pan; season with salt and pepper. Cover the pan and cook for 6 minutes.
7. Once cooked, sprinkle with cilantro.
8. Serve and enjoy!

Frittata With Feta and Green Onion

Feta frittatas are a delicious, convenient keto meal. The leftovers can be stored in your fridge for a quick and healthy meal the following day.

Time: 25 minutes

Serving Size: 2 servings

Prep Time: 10 minutes

Cook Time: 15 minutes

Nutritional Facts/Info:

Calories 203

Carbs 7 g

Fat 12 g

Protein 17 g

Ingredients:

- 1 thinly sliced green onion
- 2 large eggs, pre-beaten or whisked
- 1 minced small garlic clove
- 4 tablespoons crumbled feta cheese. Divide into 4 equal parts
- 1/2 cup egg substitute
- 4 slices of avocado, peeled and sliced thinly
- a dash of extra virgin olive oil
- 1/3 cup plum tomatoes, chopped
- 2 tablespoons sour cream, reduced-fat if preferred

Directions:

1. Preheat a well-oiled, 6-inch nonstick skillet over medium heat.
2. Add sliced onion and garlic to your skillet. Cook until soft.
3. In a mixing bowl, combine the pre-beaten eggs and 3 tablespoons of feta cheese.
4. Mix the egg and feta well..
5. Pour the egg mixture into the skillet. You should see the edges of the mixture begin to set almost immediately.
6. Cover with a lid and cook for 4-6 minutes or until nearly set.
7. Add leftover feta cheese and tomato to the skillet.
8. Cover and cook for another 2-3 minutes or until the eggs are fully cooked.
9. Let sit for 5 minutes, then cut in half and serve with sour cream and avocado.

Red and Green Frittata

Bacon and asparagus complement each other in flavor and color, and they are rich in protein! These bacon and asparagus frittatas can be stored for a convenient meal the next day.

Time: 35 minutes

Serving Size: 6 servings

Prep Time: 10 minutes

Cook Time: 25 minutes

Nutritional Facts/Info:

Calories 344

Carbs 7 g

Fat 24 g

Protein 23 g

Ingredients:

- 12 ounces bacon
- 1 cup onion, chopped
- 2 cups fresh asparagus, cut in 1/2-inch pieces
- 10 large eggs, beaten
- 2 garlic cloves, minced
- 1/2 teaspoon salt for seasoning
- 1/4 cup minced parsley
- 1 thinly sliced large tomato
- 1/4 teaspoon pepper
- 1 cup cheddar cheese, shredded

Directions:

1. Cook bacon until crisp (in a 9- or 10-inch ovenproof pan).
2. Remove bacon and crumble into pieces.
3. Drain all but 1 tablespoon of the bacon drippings.
4. On a medium-high setting, heat the drippings.
5. Sauté the asparagus, onion, and garlic until the onion is tender and translucent.
6. Put aside a third of the bacon crumbles.
7. Combine the remaining bacon, eggs, parsley, salt, and pepper in a large mixing bowl.
8. Whisk together your eggs.
9. Pour the egg mixture into the pan and stir to distribute evenly.
10. Top with tomato, cheese, and the bacon that was set aside.
11. Cover your pan and cook the contents over medium-low heat until the eggs are almost set, approximately 10-15 minutes.
12. Preheat the broiler. Broil for 2 minutes or until lightly browned. Serve straight away.

Spicey, Bacon Omelet

Spicey in flavor and rich in protein and antioxidant-rich foods, the Southwestern omelet is the perfect body fuel to start your day, and keep hunger at bay.

Time: 20 minutes

Serving Size: 4 servings

Prep Time: 10 minutes

Cook Time: 10 minutes

Nutritional Facts/Info:

Calories 390

Carbs 8 g

Fat 31 g

Protein 22 g

Ingredients:

- 1/2 cup onion, =chopped
- 1 tablespoon canola oil
- 1 minced jalapeno pepper
- 6 bacon strips, pre-cooked and diced
- 6 lightly beaten large eggs
- 1 ripe avocado, thinly sliced
- 1 chopped small tomato
- Salt and pepper for seasoning
- 1 cup shredded Monterey Jack cheese, divided into two equal parts
- Salsa, optional

Directions:

1. Heat oil in a large skillet. Cook onion and jalapeno until tender then set aside using a slotted spoon.

2. In a separate bowl, whisk together your eggs, seasoning to taste.

3. Pour the eggs into the same skillet, cover, and simmer for 3-4 minutes over low heat.

4. Add the jalapeno mixture, bacon, lettuce, avocado, and 1/2 cup cheese to half of your omelet.

5. Fold the plain side of your omelet over the half with vegetables.

6. Cook for an additional 3–4 minutes or until the eggs are done.

7. Serve omelet with salsa if desired after sprinkling with reserved cheese.

Bacon and Cheese Ham Steaks

This meat-lovers breakfast is packed with good fats that stave off hunger and help you to feel satiated after a long fast.

Time: 25 minutes

Serving Size: 4 servings

Prep Time: 10 minutes

Cook Time: 15 minutes

Nutritional Facts/Info:

Calories 352

Carbs 5 g

Fat 22 g

Protein 34 g

Ingredients:

- 2 tablespoons butter
- 1 shallot, finely chopped
- 1/2 pound sliced fresh mushrooms
- 1/8 teaspoon coarsely ground pepper
- 2 minced garlic cloves
- 1 cup Gruyere cheese, shredded
- 1 pre-cooked cooked boneless ham steak weighting around 1 pound, cut into 4 equal pieces
- 1 tablespoon fresh parsley, minced (optional)
- 4 bacon strips, pre-cooked and diced or crumbled

Directions:

1. Melt butter in a large nonstick skillet over medium-high heat.
2. Cook mushrooms and shallot, stirring often, for 4-6 minutes or until they are tender.
3. Add garlic and pepper. Cook for an additional minute.
4. Remove from the pan and set aside.
5. Clean the pan with a paper towel.
6. Add ham steak to the pan and cook on one side for 3 minutes.
7. Flip the ham over and top the cooked side with cheese and bacon.
8. Cook for another 2-4 minutes, or until the cheese has melted and the ham is well cooked.
9. Top with your mushroom and shallot mixture. Sprinkle with parsley, if desired and serve.

Cheesy French Style Omelet

Timeless and traditional, French omelets are quick and easy to make and are the perfect meal after a morning cardio workout.

Time: 20 minutes

Serving Size: 2 servings

Prep Time: 10 minutes

Cook Time: 10 minutes

Nutritional Facts/Info:

Calories 186

Carbs 4 g

Fat 9 g

Protein 22 g

Ingredients:

- 2 eggs, large
- 1/4 cup milk, skim
- 4 large egg whites
- 1/8 teaspoon pepper
- 1/8 teaspoon salt
- 1 tablespoon onion, chopped
- 1/4 cup cubed ham, pre-cooked
- 1/4 cup shredded cheddar cheese, reduced-fat (if preferred full fat)
- 1 tablespoon green pepper, chopped

Directions:

1. Over medium heat, brush a 10-inch skillet with cooking oil.
2. In a separate bowl, whisk your eggs and add seasoning to taste.
3. Pour the egg mixture into the pan. The edges of the mixture should set immediately.
4. Move cooked portions of your eggs toward the middle of the skillet, allowing uncooked eggs to flow beneath.
5. When the eggs have cooked and are no longer runny, top one half with onion, ham, pepper and cheese.
6. Fold the omelet, empty side over ingredient side into a half-moon.
7. To serve, cut in half.

Savory Sausage and Sage Patties

If you love savory flavors, these sausage patties are going to be your new go-to! A perfect breakfast for meat-lovers who don't want to compromise on big taste. The flavors of sage and onion meld together to make these patties a cut above. They can be eaten on their own or as a side.

Time: 25 minutes

Serving Size: 8 servings

Prep Time: 10 minutes

Cook Time: 15 minutes

Nutritional Facts/Info:

Calories 162

Carbs 1 g

Fat 11 g

Protein 13 g

Ingredients:

- 1 pound ground pork
- 1/4 cup buttermilk
- 3/4 cup cheddar cheese, shredded
- 2 teaspoons sage
- 1 tablespoon chopped onion
- 1 teaspoon of pepper and salt, to season
- A pinch of garlic powder and dried oregano

Directions:

1. In a medium-sized mixing bowl, combine all ingredients. Stir gently but thoroughly, taking care not to overwork the meat.
2. Using your hands, form six to eight patties to your desired thickness. Place them in the refrigerator to firm up for about an hour.
3. Cook the sausage patties in a skillet on medium heat for about eight minutes. Flip and cook for another eight minutes, or until they reach an internal temperature of 160°F.
4. Serve hot and enjoy! Try it with cheese or paired with your favorite omelet.

Popeye's Mushroom Scramble

Some days, a lighter, meat-free breakfast is what you want. These scrambled eggs made with spinach and mushrooms are a great source of protein and high in iron. They are sure to satisfy your hunger without weighing you down.

Time: 15 minutes

Serving Size: 2 servings

Prep Time: 5 minutes

Cook Time: 10 minutes

Nutritional Facts/Info:

Calories 162

Carbs 2 g

Fat 11 g

Protein 14 g

Ingredients:

- 2 eggs, large
- ⅛ teaspoon salt to season
- 2 =egg whites, large
- 1 teaspoon butter
- ⅛ teaspoon pepper to season
- ½ cup fresh baby spinach, chopped
- ½ cup mushrooms, thinly sliced fresh
- 2 tablespoons Provolone cheeses, shredded

Directions:

1. Mix the eggs, egg whites, salt, and pepper until combined.
2. Using a small nonstick skillet over medium-high heat, melt butter.
3. Add your mushrooms to the skillet on their own, stirring occasionally. Cook 3-4 minutes, until tender.
4. Add spinach and cook until wilted.
5. Bring heat down to medium.
6. Add egg mixture to the skillet with the veggies.
7. Stir constantly until the eggs are fully set and no runny egg mixture remains.
8. Add shredded cheese and fold into the scrambled eggs.
9. Heat until the cheese has melted (this usually only takes a minute or two).
10. Serve immediately.

Triple Threat Quiche Cups

You can't go wrong with broccoli, bacon, and cheese. These quiche cups have all three and 16g of protein! Make a double batch and freeze some for breakfast on-the-go or snacking.

Time: 25 minutes

Serving Size: 12 servings

Prep Time: 10 minutes

Cook Time: 15 minutes

Nutritional Facts/Info:

Calories 291

Carbs 4 g

Fat 24 g

Protein 16 g

Ingredients:

- 1 cup broccoli, fresh
- 6 large eggs, slightly beaten
- 1 cup cheese, shredded
- ½ cup bacon bits
- ¾ cup heavy whipping cream
- ¼ teaspoon salt to season
- 1 shallot, minced
- ¼ teaspoon pepper to season

Directions:

1. Preheat the oven to 350° Fahrenheit. Fill greased muffin cups halfway with broccoli and cheese.
2. In a medium mixing bowl, combine all remaining ingredients.
3. Pour the mixture on top of the broccoli and cheese in the muffin cups.
4. Bake for 15-20 minutes, or until set.

Cheesy-Greens Mediterranean Omelet

Not too keen on meat first thing in the morning? These Mediterranean broccoli and cheese omelets are rich in iron, protein, and calcium.

Time: 30 minutes

Serving Size: 4 servings

Prep Time: 15 minutes

Cook Time: 15 minutes

Nutritional Facts/Info:

Calories 230

Carbs 5 g

Fat 17 g

Protein 15 g

Ingredients:

- 2-3 cups broccoli florets, fresh
- ¼ cup milk
- 6 eggs
- Salt and pepper to taste
- ⅓ cup Greek olives, sliced, no pits
- ⅓ cup Romano cheese, grated
- 1 ½ tablespoons olive oil
- Parsley, fresh (optional)

Directions:

1. Preheat the oven to broil.

2. Place a steamer basket over 1 inch of water in a large saucepan.
3. Place broccoli in the basket.
4. Bring water to a rolling boil.
5. Reduce to low heat and steam for 4-6 minutes, until the broccoli is tender but not wilted.
6. Whisk together eggs, milk, and your preference of salt and pepper in another bowl.
7. Combine the steamed broccoli, grated cheese, and olives in a mixing bowl.
8. Heat oil in a 10-inch ovenproof skillet over medium heat, then add the egg mixture.
9. Cook for around five minutes, uncovered.
10. Broil for around three minutes, a few inches from the oven heat source, or until eggs are ready.
11. Wait five minutes before folding the omelet in half.
12. Cut your cooked omelet in half and add optional garnishes.

Smooth and Creamy Asparagus Omelet

High fiber breakfasts don't have to make you cringe. Asparagus and cream cheese take your eggs to another level while still being quick and delicious!

Time: 20 minutes

Serving Size: 2 servings

Prep Time: 10 minutes

Cook Time: 10 minutes

Nutritional Facts/Info:

Calories 350

Carbs 6 g

Fat 29 g

Protein 16 g

Ingredients:

- 4 fresh asparagus spears, trimmed and cut into 1-inch pieces
- ¼ cup sour cream
- 4 large eggs
- ¼ teaspoon salt
- 2 teaspoons dried minced onion
- 2 teaspoons butter
- ¼ teaspoon red pepper flakes, crushed
- 2 ounces cubed and softened cream cheese

Directions:

1. Boil water in a small saucepan (filled to about the ¾ mark).
2. Drop in your asparagus and cook until crisp but tender (this takes about 2-4 minutes).
3. Immerse cooked asparagus in ice water immediately. Shake off excess water and gently pat asparagus dry.
4. Combine the eggs, pepper flakes, sour cream, onion, and cinnamon.
5. Over medium-high heat, melt butter in a large nonstick skillet.
6. Pour your egg mixture into the buttered pan. The eggs should begin to set right away.
7. Using a spatula or wooden spoon, move the cooked portions to the middle and allow the runny mixture to cook around the edges.
8. When the eggs are fully cooked, turn the heat to low. On one side of your omelet, spread cream cheese and top with the asparagus spears.
9. Fold the omelet in half to cover the ingredients.
10. Cover the pan and set aside for 1-2 minutes, allowing the cream cheese to melt.
11. Cut in half and serve hot.

Keto-Friendly Spinach Quiche

While this recipe may take a little more time to prepare, bulk batches can be made and frozen for those mornings when you are short on time.

Time: 1 hour 5 minutes

Serving Size: 8 servings

Prep Time: 25 minutes

Cook Time: 40 minutes

Nutritional Facts/Info:

Calories 251

Carbs 4 g

Fat 18g

Protein 18 g

Ingredients:

- 1 cup onion, chopped
- 1 tablespoon olive, coconut, or vegetable oil
- 1 cup fresh mushrooms, thinly sliced
- ⅔ cup pre-cooked ham, diced finely
- 1 package (10 ounces) frozen spinach, pre-chopped, thawed and well-drained
- 3 cups Muenster or Monterey Jack cheese, shredded
- 5 large eggs, beaten
- ⅛ teaspoon pepper to season

Directions:

1. Heat oil in a large skillet. Add onion and mushrooms and sauté until tender.
2. Add ham and spinach, cooking until the mixture has thickened and very little liquid remains.
3. Allow to cool slightly.
4. Preheat the oven to 350 degrees Fahrenheit.
5. Combine remaining ingredients in a bowl and blend with the cooled spinach mixture.
6. Evenly fill a greased 9-inch pie dish or quiche dish with the mixture.
7. Bake until a toothpick or knife inserted in the middle comes out clean, roughly 40-45 minutes.

Greens, Eggs, and Ham

A perfect balance of meat, veggies, egg, and cheese, this flavorful dish is easy to prepare and can easily be made the night before and heated up so you can dine and dash!

Time: 30 minutes

Serving Size: 4 servings

Prep Time: 15 minutes

Cook Time: 15 minutes

Nutritional Facts/Info:

Calories 321

Carbs 4 g

Fat 23 g

Protein 26 g

Ingredients:

- 6 eggs, large
- Dash of salt to season
- ¼ teaspoon pepper
- 1 cup pre-cooked ham, cubed
- 1 ¼ cups Swiss cheese, shredded and divided
- 1 cup fresh broccoli, chopped
- 1 tablespoon butter

Directions:

1. Set the oven to broil.

2. Combine eggs, pepper, and salt. Mix in cubed ham and 1 cup of shredded cheese.
3. Over medium-high heat, melt butter in a 10-inch ovenproof skillet.
4. Cook broccoli in the skillet until soft, stirring continuously.
5. Reduce the heat to low and add your egg mixture to the skillet.
6. Cook for about 4-6 minutes, or until the eggs are almost cooked through.
7. Sprinkle the remaining ¼ cup of cheese on top.
8. Place the skillet in the oven and broil for 2-3 minutes, or until cheese has melted and eggs are cooked.
9. Remove the skillet and let it cool for roughly 5 minutes.
10. Cut into quarters and serve!

Mile High Omelet

Rich, creamy flavors in a meal that is quick to make and store, this one dish wonder is a filling meal for anyone who wakes up hungry.

Time: 30 minutes

Serving Size: 6 servings

Prep Time: 15 minutes

Cook Time: 15 minutes

Nutritional Facts/Info:

Calories 235

Carbs 4 g

Fat 16 g

Protein 17 g

Ingredients:

- 8 eggs, large
- 1 cup cheddar cheese, shredded
- ½ cup half-and-half cream
- ¼ cup green pepper, finely chopped
- 1 cup pre-cooked ham, finely chopped
- ¼ cup onion, finely chopped

Directions:

1. Preheat the oven to 400°F.
2. Whisk the eggs and cream together in a large mixing bowl.

3. Add the cheese, ham, green pepper, and onion to the egg mixture.
4. Fill a greased 9-inch square baking dish halfway with the batter.
5. Bake for 20-25 minutes, or until golden brown.

Tri-Color Scramble

With a simple ingredient list and requiring very little prep time, these scrambled eggs are the perfect solution when you find yourself in need of a quick, easy morning meal.

Time: 15 minutes

Serving Size:

Prep Time: 10 minutes

Cook Time: 5 minutes

Nutritional Facts/Info:

Calories 188

Carbs 4 g

Fat 13 g

Protein 14 g

Ingredients:

- 8 eggs, large
- ⅛ to 1/4 tsp dill weed
- ¼ cup 2% milk
- ¼ teaspoon pepper
- ¼ teaspoon salt
- ½ cup red pepper, chopped
- 1 tablespoon butter
- ½ cup, fresh tomato, chopped
- ¼ cup onion, chopped

Directions:

1. Combine eggs, dill, milk, salt, and pepper in a bowl using a whisk.
2. Melt butter in a 12-inch nonstick skillet over medium-high heat.
3. Add red pepper and onion, cooking until the onion is tender.
4. Remove the pan from the heat.
5. Pour egg mixture into the same pan; cook over medium heat, stirring occasionally until the egg thickens and begins to break apart.
6. Serve warm and enjoy!

Avo Bacon Scramble

Packed with good fats, vitamins, and minerals, avocado–when paired with protein-packed eggs–is the perfect breakfast after early morning workouts.

Time: 10 minutes

Serving Size: 6 servings

Prep Time: 5 minutes

Cook Time: 5 minutes

Nutritional Facts/Info:

Calories 233

Carbs 4 g

Fat 19 g

Protein 12 g

Ingredients:

- 8 eggs, large
- ½ teaspoon salt
- ½ cup 2% milk
- 1 medium ripe avocado, peeled and cubed
- ¼ teaspoon pepper
- 6 bacon strips, pre- cooked, diced or crumbled
- 2 tablespoons butter

Directions:

1. Whisk eggs together in a large mixing bowl.
2. Add the cream, salt, and pepper to your egg mixture.

3. Melt butter in a pan over medium heat.
4. Add the egg mixture to the pan and cook, stirring continuously, until the eggs are fully set.
5. Sprinkle crispy bacon on top, and serve on a bed of avocado. Add another level of flavor by folding in some shredded cheese while it's still hot!

Rustic Apple-Turkey Sausage Patties

Easy to make and packed full of flavor, these sausages are a great meal add-on and are sure to please a crowd of any size around your table! You can swap out turkey for ground chicken as well!

Time: 25 minutes

Serving Size: 8 servings

Prep Time: 10 minutes

Cook Time: 15 minutes

Nutritional Facts/Info:

Calories 92

Carbs 4 g

Fat 5 g

Protein 9 g

Ingredients:

- 1 large granny smith apple, peeled and diced
- 1 teaspoon salt to season
- 2 teaspoons poultry seasoning
- 1 pound ground turkey
- ¼ teaspoon pepper

Directions:

1. Combine seasonings and apples in a large mixing bowl.
2. Add the ground turkey and stir well.
3. Use the mixture to create eight 3-inch patties.

4. Cook patties over medium heat for 5-6 minutes on each side (until no longer pink) in a large, greased cast-iron pan, or another heavy skillet.
5. Remove from heat and place on a paper towel-lined plate. Let sit for 5 minutes.
6. Serve and enjoy.

Swiss Cheese "Zittata"

Zoodles and zaghetti are popular zucchini-based pasta substitutes, so why not try a zucchini-filled frittata? Delicate, delicious, and creamy, these Zucchini Frittatas are an amazing crustless quiche without the carbs.

Time: 20 minutes

Serving Size: 2 servings

Prep Time: 10 minutes

Cook Time: 10 minutes

Nutritional Facts/Info:

Calories 261

Carbs 7 g

Fat 18 g

Protein 18 g

Ingredients:

- 3 eggs, large
- 1 teaspoon canola oil
- ¼ teaspoon salt to season
- 1 cup zucchini, , coarsely shredded
- ½ cup onion, chopped
- Coarsely ground pepper
- ½ cup Swiss cheese, shredded

Directions:

1. Preheat the oven to 350 degrees Fahrenheit.

2. Whisk the eggs and salt in a mixing bowl.
3. Heat oil over medium heat in an 8-inch ovenproof skillet sprayed with cooking spray.
4. Sauté zucchini and onion until tender-crisp, around 8 minutes.
5. Add the egg mixture to the pan and simmer for 5-6 minutes, or until almost set.
6. Sprinkle the top with cheese before baking for 4-5 minutes uncovered, until the cheese is melted.
7. Season with pepper, if desired, and serve.

Two-Bite Breakfast Bakes

Quick, easy, and delightfully delicious for those who prefer to plan ahead and have a healthy, iron rich breakfast ready to go as soon as their feet hit the floor. Bake ahead and enjoy!

Time: 30 minutes

Serving Size: 24 servings

Prep Time: 10 minutes

Cook Time: 20 minutes

Nutritional Facts/Info:

Calories 128

Carbs 4 g

Fat 9 g

Protein 10 g

Ingredients:

- 1 cup whole-milk ricotta cheese, grated
- ⅔ cup fresh mushrooms, chopped
- ¾ cup Parmesan cheese, finely grated
- 1 egg, large
- 1 package (10 ounces) frozen chopped spinach, thawed and squeezed dry
- ¼ teaspoon salt to season
- ½ teaspoon dried oregano
- 24 slices pepperoni
- ¼ teaspoon pepper to season

Directions:

1. Preheat the oven to 375 degrees Fahrenheit.
2. Whisk egg in a bowl.
3. Mix in the mushrooms, spinach, salt, oregano, and pepper.
4. Place a pepperoni slice at the base of each of your greased mini-muffin cups.
5. Add a thin layer of grated cheese on top of each pepperoni slice.
6. Fill each cup to three-quarters full with your premixed ingredients.
7. Bake for 20-25 minutes, or until the center is fully baked.
8. To free frittatas, carefully run a knife along the edges of muffin cups.

Frittata Italiana

A firm Italian favorite, this frittata serves as a filling, flavorful, and healthy meal, making it a brunch must-have!

Time: 30 minutes

Serving Size: 4 servings

Prep Time: 15 minutes

Cook Time: 15 minutes

Nutritional Facts/Info:

Calories 176

Carbs 4 g

Fat 11 g

Protein 15 g

Ingredients:

- 6 egg whites, large
- ½ teaspoon dried oregano
- 3 whole eggs, large
- ¼ teaspoon salt to season
- ¼ teaspoon pepper to season
- ¼ teaspoon garlic powder
- 1 tablespoon olive oil
- ¼ cup sweet red pepper, finely chopped
- 1 small onion, finely chopped
- 1 cup fresh baby spinach
- 2 turkey bacon strips, diced
- ½ cup part-skim mozzarella cheese, shredded
- 3 tablespoons fresh basil leaves, thinly sliced

Directions:

1. Preheat the oven to broil.
2. Whisk together the eggs, egg whites, and spices in a large mixing bowl.
3. Heat the oil over medium-high heat in an 8-inch ovenproof skillet.
4. Add onions to the heated pan and cook until fragrant.
5. Add red pepper and bacon to your pre-cooked onions, and cook to the desired level of tenderness (tender-crisp is recommended).
6. Reduce to a medium-low heat setting and top with spinach, cooking until the spinach is wilted.
7. Pour the egg mixture into the pan.
8. Cook until eggs are nearly thickened, moving cooked portions toward the middle and allowing uncooked eggs to flow beneath.
9. Remove from heat and top with basil and cheese.
10. Broil for 2-3 minutes or until the eggs are fully set.
11. Let cool for 5 minutes before cutting into quarters and serve!

The Cheesy Classic

Cheese and chives are a culinary favorite and, when added to your breakfast omelet, this dynamic duo create the taste of summer all year round.

Time: 15 minutes

Serving Size: 2 servings

Prep Time: 10 minutes

Cook Time: 5 minutes

Nutritional Facts/Info:

Calories 216

Carbs 1 g

Fat 18 g

Protein 13 g

Ingredients:

- 3 eggs, large
- 2 tablespoons water
- 1 tablespoon fresh chives, minced
- Salt and pepper to season
- ¼ to ½ cup cheddar cheese, shredded
- 1 tablespoon butter

Directions:

1. Melt butter in a small nonstick skillet over medium-high heat.

2. Whisk together eggs, water, salt, and pepper in a small bowl. Add the chives and mix well.
3. Pour the egg mixture into the pan. The edges of the mixture should set immediately.
4. Push cooked portions toward the middle as the eggs set, allowing uncooked eggs to flow beneath.
5. When the eggs are fully cooked, sprinkle cheese on one half and fold. Serve and enjoy.

Rainbow Frittata

The addition of eggs to this filling vegetable-based breakfast makes it perfect for those post-workout hunger pangs. A wide variety of veggies lend their colors (and flavors) to this dish, hence the name. Make sure you have extras if you aren't dining alone or your guests are sure to be green with envy.

Time: 45 minutes

Serving Size: 8 servings

Prep Time: 25 minutes

Cook Time: 20 minutes

Nutritional Facts/Info:

Calories 130

Carbs 5 g

Fat 8 g

Protein 9 g

Ingredients:

- 8 eggs, large
- 2 tablespoons lemon juice
- ½ cup whole-milk ricotta cheese
- ¼ teaspoon pepper to season
- ½ teaspoon salt to season
- 1 package (8 ounces) frozen asparagus spears, thawed
- 1 tablespoon olive oil
- ½ cup sweet red and/or green pepper, finely chopped
- 1 large onion, thinly sliced and halved
- ¼ cup baby portobello mushrooms, sliced

Directions:

1. Preheat the oven to 350 degrees Fahrenheit.
2. Heat the oil in a 10-inch ovenproof skillet over medium heat.
3. Remove 8 asparagus spears from the package and set them aside. Chop remaining asparagus into 1-inch pieces.
4. Add chopped asparagus, onion, red pepper, and mushrooms to the pan, cooking until the mushrooms are tender.
5. Whisk together the first five ingredients in a large mixing bowl. Add whisked egg ingredients to your vegetables. Place the skillet in the oven and bake for 20-25 minutes.
6. Remove from the oven and arrange the set-aside asparagus spears on top of the eggs to mimic wheel spokes.
7. Return to the oven and bake for another 5 minutes.
8. Cut into wedges to serve.

Bacon Wrapped Egg Bites

Convenient to freeze and store for an on-the-go meal, these bacon and egg bites are for those who like to multitask in the morning.

Time: 35 minutes

Serving Size: 6 servings

Prep Time: 20 minutes

Cook Time: 15 minutes

Nutritional Facts/Info:

Calories 311

Carbs 1 g

Fat 28 g

Protein 13 g

Ingredients:

- Between 12 and 18 strips of bacon
- 6 eggs, large
- 1 teaspoon butter
- Fresh ground pepper to season

Directions:

1. Preheat the oven to 325 degrees Fahrenheit.
2. Cook bacon in a large skillet over medium heat until it is cooked but still floppy.
3. Dab excess grease from the bacon using paper towels. Cut your bacon strips in half.

4. Lightly grease muffin cups.
5. Line each muffin cup with 2-4 bacon strips, making sure to overlap each piece.
6. Crack an egg into each bacon-lined muffin cup.
7. Bake for 12-18 minutes, or until the whites are fully set and the yolks are thickening but not firm. Season with pepper, if desired.

Chapter 4: Keto Lunch Recipes

For some, the thought of eating a large meal at the beginning of the day is not appealing. If you are one of those people, your main caloric intake should occur at lunchtime. Depending on your intermittent fasting protocol, your lunch should be eaten at around noon. Below are rich, flavorful meals that help to satisfy your hunger and assist in balancing sugar levels after long fasting periods.

Having two large meals per day can help to keep calorie intakes correct by ensuring that you are not snacking excessively. If you prefer to work out in the afternoon, a large lunch will provide you with the energy needed to get through your exercise routine without an energy slump.

It is important to remember that, when fasting for longer periods, lunch should only be skipped on 24 hour fasting days, or if a large breakfast has been eaten. Choosing to eat a larger breakfast, skipping lunch, and eating a satiating supper is advisable for those who do not exercise in the afternoon.

Simple Cauli-Floret Mac'n Cheese

An easy-to-make low-carb meal with rich, cheesy, and creamy flavors. This keto-friendly, vegetarian version of a lunchtime favorite will curb your cravings for pasta.

Time: 40 minutes

Serving Size: 4 servings

Prep Time: 15 minutes

Cook Time: 25 minutes

Nutritional Facts/Info:

Calories 389

Carbs 9.5 g

Fat 35 g

Protein 12 g

Ingredients:

- 1 head cauliflower, cut into bite-sized pieces
- 1 teaspoon mixed herbs
- 1 teaspoon salt
- 3 tablespoons olive/canola oil
- ½ teaspoon freshly ground black pepper
- ½ cup heavy whipping cream
- 1 cup cheddar cheese, shredded ('old' recommended)
- 1 pinch ground nutmeg
- 1 tablespoon ghee
- 3 tablespoons Parmesan cheese, grated

Directions:

1. Preheat the oven to 450 degrees.
2. Use aluminum foil to line a baking sheet.
3. In a bowl, drizzle cauliflower with oil and toss until the cauliflower is evenly coated.
4. Place cauliflower on the baking sheet. Spread evenly. Sprinkle it with salt, pepper, and mixed herbs to taste.
5. Place in the oven and roast for approximately 10-15 minutes, or until crisp.
6. In a saucepan, over medium heat, mix the Cheddar cheese, heavy cream, ghee, and nutmeg. Cook for 5 minutes, until bubbling.
7. In an 8-inch baking dish, combine the cooked cauliflower and sauce. Mix to coat well.
8. Cover with a sprinkling of Parmesan.
9. Bake for 10 minutes or until golden.

Keto Beef Egg Roll in a Bowl

A fast, easy, keto meal that can be prepped for a meal on the go. Not keen on beef? You can substitute another lean protein for the red meat in this recipe.

Time: 30 minutes

Serving Size: 6 servings

Prep Time: 15 minutes

Cook Time: 15 minutes

Nutritional Facts/Info:

Calories 350

Carbs 12 g

Fat 24 g

Protein 20.6 g

Ingredients:

- 2 tablespoons sesame oil
- 5 green onions, chopped (separate the white and green parts)
- ½ cup onion, diced
- 1 ½ pounds ground beef
- 3 cloves garlic, minced
- ½ teaspoon ground ginger
- 1 tablespoon chili-garlic sauce (like sriracha)
- Ground black pepper and sea salt to season
- 3 tablespoons soy sauce
- 1, 14 ounce packaged coleslaw mix
- 1 tablespoon apple cider vinegar

Directions:

1. Over medium-high heat, heat the oil in a large skillet.
2. Add the white parts of green onion, diced onion and garlic to the pan.
3. Cook approximately 5 minutes until garlic is fragrant and onions are transparent.
4. In a bowl, combine the ground beef, sriracha, ginger, salt, and black pepper. Add to pan.
5. Cook the beef until brown and crumbly, approximately 5 minutes.
6. Drain fat from cooked ground beef, if necessary. Then, in a large mixing bowl, combine the ground beef, coleslaw blend, soy sauce, and apple cider vinegar.
7. Return to pan, cook for another 4 minutes, removing from heat before the coleslaw is wilted.
8. If desired, sprinkle with the green part of the chopped green onions.
9. Serve and enjoy!

Cobb Salad

Cobb salad is an American favorite and is the perfect addition to your weekend barbeque menu.

Time: 50 minutes

Serving Size: 6 servings

Prep Time: 20 minutes

Cook Time: 30 minutes

Nutritional Facts/Info:

Calories 267

Carbs 10.2 g

Fat 39.9 g

Protein 31.7 g

Ingredients:

- 6 slices bacon
- 1 head iceberg lettuce, shredded
- 3 eggs, large
- 2 tomatoes, seeded and chopped
- 3 cups chicken meat, cooked and cut into bite-sized pieces
- 1 avocado - peeled, pitted, and diced
- ¾ cup blue cheese, crumbled
- 1, 8 ounce bottle Ranch-style salad dressing
- 3 green onions, finely chopped

Directions:

1. Add cold water to a small pot (fill approximately halfway) and add the eggs.
2. Over medium-high heat, bring water to a boil. Allow eggs to cook for 6 minutes.
3. Remove pot from heat and set aside (leave the eggs in the water) for 10 to 12 minutes.
4. Remove the eggs from the water. Let sit until they are cool enough to peel and chop.
5. In a large, deep skillet, over medium-high heat cook the bacon until uniformly browned.
6. Drain the bacon. Then slice or crumble the bacon onto a separate plate.
7. Place shredded lettuce on six individual plates.
8. On top of each lettuce bed, evenly divide and arrange the chicken, eggs, tomatoes, blue cheese, bacon, avocado, and green onions.
9. Drizzle with your favorite vinaigrette and serve.

Classic Shrimp Scampi with Keto Broccoli 'Noodles'

To keep this recipe keto-friendly, the pasta is replaced with flavorful broccoli noodles. Seasoning with cheese and herbs will add an extra kick to the dish!

Time: 30 minutes

Serving Size: 4 servings

Prep Time: 15 minutes

Cook Time: 15 minutes

Nutritional Facts/Info:

Calories 267

Carbs 12.8 g

Fat 14.2 g

Protein 23.5 g

Ingredients:

- 2 large heads of broccoli with long stems
- Black pepper (ground) and salt, to season
- 2 tablespoons olive oil, equally divided
- 1 pound raw peeled, cleaned and deveined, shrimp
- 2 cloves minced garlic, minced
- 2 tablespoons lemon juice
- 2 tablespoons dry white wine
- 1 tablespoon minced fresh basil
- 2 tablespoons butter
- ½ teaspoon red pepper, crushed
- 1 tablespoon fresh chives, chopped

Directions:

1. Remove the broccoli florets from the stems. Set aside. Trim the broccoli stems.
2. Using a vegetable peeler, remove any big large 'knots' from stems.
3. Using the smallest spiralizer comb, cut into noodle-shaped strips.
4. Heat 1 tablespoon of olive oil in a large skillet, over medium-high heat.
5. Add the broccoli 'noodles' to the pan, seasoning to taste. Cook for 3 minutes.
6. Remove the pan from the heat and set it aside.
7. In a separate pan, heat the remaining olive oil and add garlic. Cook for about a minute.
8. Add the shrimp and cook for approximately 3 minutes per side, or until the shrimp are opaque.
9. Remove the shrimp from heat, placing them in a separate bowl.
10. In the same pan, combine the rest of the ingredients. Whisk constantly for 3 minutes over medium heat.
11. Return shrimp to the skillet and gently toss to coat in the wine, butter, and herb sauce.
12. Divide noodles equally into 4 bowls.
13. Serve your cooked and coated shrimp on the bed of broccoli noodles.

Portobello Pizza Pies

All the flavors of your favorite pizza minus the carbs! This quick and easy Keto-friendly meal can be eaten as a main meal or as a light lunchtime calorie top-up.

Time: 40 minutes

Serving Size: 1 serving

Prep Time: 15 minutes

Cook Time: 25 minutes

Nutritional Facts/Info:

Calories 235

Carbs 10.6 g

Fat 13.6 g

Protein 18.8 g

Ingredients:

- 1 large portobello mushroom, stem removed
- ½ cup mozzarella cheese, shredded
- 1 tablespoon spaghetti sauce
- 4 slices pepperoni sausage
- ½ tablespoon black olives, sliced
- 1 clove garlic, chopped

Directions:

1. Preheat the oven to 375 degrees.
2. Remove the stems from your mushroom, placing the mushroom cap on a baking sheet.

3. Bake for 5 minutes.
4. Remove the mushroom cap from the oven and spoon spaghetti sauce into the center.
5. Add cheese, olives, pepperoni, and garlic on top of the spaghetti sauce.
6. Cook for another 20 minutes, or until the cheese has melted and turned golden.

Easy Cheesy Keto Beef Bowls

Using fresh low-carb ingredients, our beef bowls are as tasty as any takeaway version of this all-time favorite lunch meal.

Time: 50 minutes

Serving Size: 4 servings

Prep Time: 20 minutes

Cook Time: 30 minutes

Nutritional Facts/Info:

Calories 676

Carbs 9.7 g

Fat 52.6 g

Protein 40.7 g

Ingredients:

- 2 cups cheddar cheese, shredded
- ½ package taco seasoning mix
- 1 pound ground beef
- ¼ teaspoon ground black pepper to season
- ½ teaspoon salt to season

SUGGESTED TOPPING

- 1 cup lettuce, shredded
- 1 avocado, diced
- ½ cup tomatoes, diced
- ½ cup cheddar cheese, shredded

Directions:

1. Preheat the oven to 350 degrees.
2. Cover two baking sheets with parchment paper.
3. Create four 6-inch circles of cheddar cheese on a baking sheet. Space them approximately 2 inches apart.
4. Place in the oven for 6 to 8 minutes, until the cheese melts and just begins to turn brown.
5. Remove from the oven and allow to cool for 2 to 3 minutes before gently lifting with a spatula. The cheese should still be malleable.
6. While the cheese is cooling, cover four small bowls in aluminum foil, laying them upside down on a flat surface, and drape each circle of cheese over a foil-covered cup. A bowl shape should form. Set aside to cool.
7. Place beef in a skillet over medium-high heat, cooking until browned.
8. Season to taste and cook for 1 minute more.
9. Grab your cheese bowls and fill halfway with beef mixture.
10. Add spoonfuls of toppings to your taco bowls as desired.
11. Serve and enjoy!

Pescatarian Surf 'N' Turf

Perfect for hot summer days, and an easy to assemble meal, these Seafood Stuffed Avocados are a winner among seafood lovers.

Time: 15 minutes

Serving Size: 2 servings

Prep Time: 15 minutes

Cook Time: 0 minutes

Nutritional Facts/Info:

Calories 283

Carbs 10 g

Fat 21.1 g

Protein 16.5 g

Ingredients:

- ½ cup cooked crabmeat, flaked
- 2 tablespoons cucumber, peeled and diced
- ½ cup small shrimp, cooked
- 1 teaspoon fresh parsley, chopped
- 1 tablespoon mayonnaise
- 1 pinch ground black pepper to taste
- 1 pinch salt to taste
- 1 avocado
- 1 pinch paprika

Directions:

1. Combine the crab, shrimp, cucumber, mayonnaise, and parsley in a mixing bowl.
2. Add salt and pepper to taste.
3. Toss ingredients in the bowl until well coated with spices and mayonnaise.
4. Cover and chill in the refrigerator.
5. Slice your avocado in half, removing the pit.
6. Cover the hollowed pit centers of the avocado halves with the seafood mixture.
7. Top with paprika.

Keto-Friendly Tuna Salad

A quick and easy salad, packed full of healthy fats, oils, vitamins, and minerals.

Time: 15 minutes

Serving Size: 4 servings

Prep Time: 15 minutes

Nutritional Facts/Info:

Calories 423

Carbs 6.2 g

Fat 22.8 g

Protein 46.9 g

Ingredients:

- 2 (6 ounce) drained cans water-packed tuna
- ¾ cup olive oil mayonnaise (reduced fat)
- 2 (6 ounce) cans drained olive oil-packed tuna
- juice of ½ a lime
- 2 chopped stalks celery
- salt and ground black pepper to taste to season
- ¼ chopped red onion
- 2 tbsp mustard

Directions:

1. In a large mixing bowl, combine all.
2. Toss the ingredients, ensuring everything is mixed well.
3. Serve and enjoy.

Winter's Afternoon Spaghetti Squash

Perfect for a winter afternoon, this wholesome keto meal is rich in complementary flavors to suit the most refined pallets.

Time: 1 hour 15 minutes

Serving Size: 2 servings

Prep Time: 15 minutes

Cook Time: 1 hour

Nutritional Facts/Info:

Calories 339

Carbs 20.6 g

Fat 24.3 g

Protein 13.5 g

Ingredients:

- 1 spaghetti squash, small
- salt and ground black pepper to season
- 1 tablespoon olive oil
- 4 ounces mushrooms, sliced
- 4 slices bacon, diced
- 2 cups baby spinach
- 1 clove minced garlic
- 2 tablespoons blue cheese, crumbled
- ¼ cup sour cream

Directions:

1. Use aluminum foil to line a baking sheet.

2. Preheat the oven to 400 degrees.
3. Using a sharp knife, remove the stem of the spaghetti squash.
4. After slicing the squash in half lengthwise, scrape the seeds out with a spoon.
5. Brush the squash with olive oil. Season inside with salt and pepper.
6. Bake for 45 minutes or until tender.
7. Place bacon in a broad skillet over medium-high heat, rotating regularly, for 5 to 6 minutes or until evenly browned.
8. Add mushrooms and garlic to the skillet and cook for an additional 4 to 5 minutes.
9. Add spinach to the skillet and cook until wilted.
10. Remove squash from oven. Carefully scoop out the cooked squash flesh and place it in a large mixing bowl.
11. Place the outer shells of the spaghetti squash back onto the baking sheet.
12. Place the bacon and vegetable mixture into the bowl of squash flesh, stirring well until mixed thoroughly.
13. Spoon the mixture into your squash shells until they are 3/4 full.
14. Combine the sour cream, salt, and pepper in a mixing bowl.
15. Lightly drizzle the sour cream over your filled squash shells.
16. Sprinkle with blue cheese and return to the oven, baking for another 4 to 5 minutes or until the cheese has melted and the squash has cooked through.

Not-So-Starchy Risotto

Craving starchy risotto? Our cauliflower risotto satisfies those cravings, leaving you feeling full and ready to hit the gym.

Time: 30 minutes

Serving Size: 4 servings

Prep Time: 15 minutes

Cook Time: 14 minutes

Nutritional Facts/Info:

Calories 350

Carbs 11.8 g

Fat 29.8 g

Protein 12.1 g

Ingredients:

- ¼ cup ghee
- 1 clove minced garlic
- ½ an onion, finely chopped
- 1 cup fresh mushrooms, sliced
- 1 small grated head of cauliflower
- 1 cup Parmesan cheese, grated
- ½ cup heavy whipping cream
- ¼ teaspoon ground black pepper to season
- ½ teaspoon salt to season
- ¼ teaspoon ground nutmeg

Directions:

1. In a pan, melt the ghee over medium heat.
2. Add onions and garlic. Cook for 3 minutes or until onion and garlic are tender.
3. Add the grated cauliflower and cook for a further 3 minutes.
4. Add mushrooms to the skillet, cooking the mixture until the mushrooms are soft, approximately 3 minutes.
5. In a separate skillet, mix the heavy cream, parmesan cheese, salt, pepper, and nutmeg on medium to low heat, stirring periodically until smooth, around 5 to 7 minutes.
6. Drizzle sauce on your cauliflower and mushroom risotto.
7. Serve and enjoy!

Sweet and Savory Chicken Lettuce Wraps

A quick easy summer meal that can be added to your barbeque or picnic menu, these Chicken Wraps are tasty as well as healthy.

Time: 25 minutes

Serving Size: 6 servings

Prep Time: 15 minutes

Cook Time: 10 minutes

Nutritional Facts/Info:

Calories 297

Carbs 22.8 g

Fat 12.7 g

Protein 24.4 g

Ingredients:

- 2 tablespoons canola oil
- 1 tablespoon fresh ginger root, minced
- 1 ¼ pound skinless, boneless chicken breast halves, shredded or cubed
- 2 tablespoons teriyaki sauce
- 2 tablespoons rice vinegar
- 1 pound pitted and halved dark sweet cherries
- 1 tablespoon honey
- ½ cup green onion, chopped
- 1 ½ cups carrots, shredded
- 12 lettuce leaves
- ⅓ cup sliced almonds, toasted

Directions:

1. In a large skillet, heat 1 tablespoon oil over medium-high heat.

2. Add chicken and ginger to the oil. Fry for approximately 7 to 10 minutes, or until chicken is cooked through.

3. Remove from the pan and set aside.

4. In a mixing bowl, combine the vinegar, teriyaki sauce, remaining 1 tablespoon oil, and honey. Mix until the ingredients are combined well.

5. Pour your dressing over your chicken, and add cherries, tomatoes, green onion, and almonds.

6. Evenly distribute the chicken and cherry mixture, spooning into the middle of each lettuce leaf; roll the lettuce leaf around the filling and serve.

Korean Beef and Rice for Keto

This dish can be eaten at lunch or dinner time to refuel your body after long fasting periods, or simply to curb your craving for Asian food.

Time: 40 minutes

Serving Size: 4 servings

Prep Time: 10 minutes

Cook Time: 10 minutes

Nutritional Facts/Info:

Calories 297

Carbs 8.9 g

Fat 19.1 g

Protein 22.4 g

Ingredients:

- 2 teaspoons sesame oil
- 3 cloves minced garlic
- 1 pound lean ground beef
- 1 tablespoon coconut sugar
- ¼ cup soy sauce
- ¼ teaspoon ground black pepper to season
- ¼ teaspoon ground ginger
- 2 tablespoons green onions, chopped
- 2 cups pre-packaged cauliflower rice
- 1 tablespoon sesame seeds (optional)

Directions:

1. In a big skillet, heat sesame oil over medium-high heat.
2. Add garlic and allow to fry until fragrant.
3. Add ground beef to your skillet and cook until the meat is browned and crumbly.
4. In a mixing bowl, whisk together the soy sauce, coconut sugar, ginger, and black pepper.
5. Pour over the ground beef and allow to cook for a further 3 minutes, removing the skillet from the heat when the sauce thickens.
6. Serve over cauliflower rice with green onions and sesame seeds sprinkled on top.

Fast-Breaking Chili

Rich in calories, this fast breaking chili recipe is great for after a 24 hour fast.

Time: 6 hours 35 minutes

Serving Size: 8 servings

Prep Time: 20 minutes

Cook Time: 6 hours 15 minutes

Nutritional Facts/Info:

Calories 357

Carbs 12.2 g

Fat 22 g

Protein 27.4 g

Ingredients:

- 2 pounds ground pork
- 14.5 ounce can well-drained, diced tomatoes
- 8 thick slices bacon, diced or crumbled
- 3 small finely chopped green bell peppers
- 1 finely chopped onion
- 1.25 ounce package of chili seasoning
- 6 ounce can tomato paste
- 1 pinch each of: onion powder, garlic powder, and cayenne pepper to season

Directions:

1. Add tomatoes, green bell pepper, and tomato paste to the slow cooker.
2. Stir in the spice packet, garlic powder, onion powder, salt, pepper, and cayenne pepper.
3. Heat a skillet over medium heat.
4. Add ground pork, seasoning with salt and pepper. Allow to cook for 5 to 7 minutes, or until browned and crumbly.
5. Drain and dispose of the grease from your skillet.
6. Place the pork in a slow cooker.
7. In the same skillet, add the bacon, frying for 10 minutes or until evenly browned.
8. Drain and dispose of the bacon grease.
9. Add the bacon to the slow cooker. Stir to combine.
10. Cook on low for 6 hours.

Avocados Con Taco

The addition of avocado to this all-time favorite recipe increases calories which makes it perfect for those who prefer to eat their first meal at lunch.

Time: 25 minutes

Serving Size: 4 servings

Prep Time: 10 minutes

Cook Time: 15 minutes

Nutritional Facts/Info:

Calories 785

Carbs 28.9 g

Fat 57.1 g

Protein 45 g

Ingredients:

- 4 small avocados, ripe
- 1 tablespoon extra-virgin olive oil
- Juice of 1 lime
- 1 pound ground beef
- 1 chopped medium onion
- Kosher salt
- 1 packet taco seasoning
- ⅔ cup Mexican cheese, grated
- Freshly ground black pepper to season
- ½ cup grape tomatoes, quartered
- ½ cup lettuce, shredded
- Sour cream to serve

Directions:

1. Slice the avocados into halves and remove the pits.
2. Create a bigger well by scooping out a bit of avocado with a spoon.
3. Dice the removed avocado then splash with lime juice to prevent browning. Set it aside to use later.
4. Heat oil in a medium skillet over medium heat.
5. Add onions to the skillet, stirring occasionally, until the onion is soft.
6. Add the beef to your skillet along with the taco seasoning. Use a slotted spoon, wooden spoon, or another kitchen utensil to break clumps.
7. Season beef with salt and pepper to taste.
8. When the beef is cooked through and there is no pink remaining, remove the pan from heat. Drain any grease.
9. Fill each avocado piece halfway with beef, then top with cheese, lettuce, tomato, and a dollop of sour cream.

Buffalo Shrimp Lettuce Wraps

Light but filling, our wraps are a seafood lover's favorite summer meal.

Time: 35 minutes

Serving Size: 4 servings

Prep Time: 15 minutes

Cook Time: 20 minutes

Nutritional Facts/Info:

Calories 265

Carbs 9 g

Fat 11.5 g

Protein 31.7 g

Ingredients:

- ¼ tablespoon butter
- ¼ cup hot sauce
- 2 garlic cloves, minced
- 1 pound shrimp peeled and deveined with tails removed
- 1 tablespoon extra virgin olive oil
- Freshly ground black pepper to season
- Kosher salt to season
- ¼ finely chopped red onion
- 1 head romaine, leaves separated, to serving
- ½ cup blue cheese, crumbled
- 1 thinly sliced rib of celery

Directions:

1. Melt butter in a small saucepan over medium heat.
2. Once the butter has fully melted, add the garlic and simmer for 1 minute or until fragrant.
3. Stir in the hot sauce until it is well mixed.
4. Reduce the heat to low, allow to simmer.
5. In a separate skillet, heat oil over medium heat.
6. Add shrimp to the skillet and season with salt and pepper.
7. When the sides of the shrimp turn pink, after about 2 minutes, turn them.
8. Remove the shrimp from the heat. Add sauce to shrimp.
9. Lay a large lettuce leaf on a plate and spoon shrimp into the center of the leaf. Add red onion, celery, and blue cheese before rolling into a wrap.

Broccoli Salad for Keto

Wanting to add Keto salads to your family gatherings or summer barbeque menu? This Broccoli Salad is quick and easy to make and is healthy to boot.

Time: 35 minutes

Serving Size: 4 servings

Prep Time: 15 minutes

Cook Time: 20 minutes

Nutritional Facts/Info:

Calories 320

Carbs 16.6 g

Fat 23.4 g

Protein 12.5 g

Ingredients:

FOR THE SALAD

- Kosher salt
- ½ cup cheddar cheese, shredded
- 3 heads broccoli, chopped or broken into bite-size pieces
- ¼ cup sliced almonds, toasted
- ¼ thinly sliced red onion
- 2 tablespoons fresh chives, chopped
- 3 slices bacon, cooked and cubed

FOR THE DRESSING

- 2/3 cup mayonnaise

- 1 tablespoon Dijon mustard
- 3 tablespoons apple cider vinegar
- Freshly ground black pepper to season
- Salt to season

Directions:

1. In a medium pot, bring 6 cups of salted water to a boil.
2. In a large bowl, prepare ice water as you wait for the water to heat.
3. Once the water comes to a boil, add broccoli florets and cook for 1 to 2 minutes or until tender.
4. Remove with a slotted spoon and put in the ice water bath.
5. Drain florets in a colander and set them aside.
6. Whisk together the dressing ingredients in a medium mixing bowl. Season with salt and pepper to taste.
7. Combine all the salad ingredients in a salad bowl and pour over the dressing.
8. Toss until all of the ingredients are evenly covered in the dressing.
9. Place in the refrigerator until ready to eat.

Keto-Friendly Egg Salad

Another summer barbeque favorite, our Keto-Friendly Egg Salad is an easy and versatile addition to your daily calorie intake.

Time: 25 minutes

Serving Size: 4 servings

Prep Time: 15 minutes

Cook Time: 10 minutes

Nutritional Facts/Info:

Calories 268

Carbs 8.1 g

Fat 22.1 g

Protein 11.2 g

Ingredients:

- 3 tablespoon mayonnaise
- 1 tablespoon chives, finely chopped
- 2 teaspoon lemon juice
- Salt to season
- Freshly ground black pepper to season
- 1 small avocado, cubed
- 6 peeled and chopped hard-boiled eggs
- Cooked bacon, crumbled
- Lettuce, to serve
- Paprika, optional

Directions:

1. Whisk together mayonnaise, lemon juice, and chives in a medium mixing bowl.
2. Add salt and pepper to taste.
3. Add eggs and avocado. Mix gently.
4. Before serving, toss with lettuce and bacon and top with paprika, if desired.

Bacon Sushi Rolls

All of the smoky flavors of bacon sushi without the starchy, damaging rice, these bacon sushi rolls are easy to pack for an on the go, or as a take to the office meal.

Time: 30 minutes

Serving Size: 12 servings

Prep Time: 10 minutes

Cook Time: 20 minutes

Nutritional Facts/Info:

Calories 126

Carbs 3.5 g

Fat 10.6 g

Protein 4.6 g

Ingredients

- 6 halved slices bacon
- 2 thinly sliced, medium carrots
- 2 thinly sliced Persian or pickling cucumbers
- 4 ounces softened cream cheese
- 1 small, sliced avocado
- Sesame seeds to garnish if desired

Directions:

1. Cover a baking sheet with aluminum foil.
2. Preheat the oven to 400 degrees.

3. Place bacon halves evenly on the baking sheet. Bake for 12 minutes, or until mildly crisp but still pliable.

4. Cut carrots, avocado and cucumbers into pieces the approximate thickness of the bacon.

5. Divide cream cheese evenly between bacon slices. Spread a layer of cream cheese on each slice, once cooled.

6. Starting on one end, pack the vegetables tightly and roll the bacon to create your sushi.

7. Serve with sesame seeds as a garnish.

Fat Bomb Burger Bites

Delicious buttery flavors that will keep you feeling fuller for longer, these bite-sized, meaty treats are great for a post-workout or road trip meal.

Time: 30 minutes

Serving Size: 20 servings

Prep Time: 15 minutes

Cook Time: 15 minutes

Nutritional Facts/Info:

Calories 80

Carbs 0 g

Fat 7 g

Protein 5 g

Ingredients:

- Cooking spray
- 1/2 teaspoon garlic powder
- 1 pound ground beef
- Freshly ground black pepper to season
- Salt to season
- 2 ounces cheddar cheese, cut into 20 pieces
- 2 tablespoons cold butter, cut into 20 pieces

TO SERVE

- Tomatoes, thinly sliced
- Lettuce leaves

- 1 teaspoon mustard

Directions:

1. Preheat the oven to 375 degrees.
2. Coat the cups of a mini muffin pan with cooking spray.
3. Evenly mix beef with garlic powder, salt, and pepper in a medium bowl.
4. Spoon 1 teaspoon of beef into the bottom of each muffin cup, being sure it is even.
5. Place a slice of butter on top, then use another teaspoon of beef top sandwich the butter.
6. In each cup, place a slice of cheddar on top of the meat, then press the remaining beef on top.
7. Bake for 15 minutes, or until the meat is well done.
8. Allow to cool slightly before serving.
9. We suggest using a spatula to carefully remove each burger from the tin.
10. Serve on a bed of lettuce and tomatoes with mustard on the side.

Winter Asian Beef Salad With a Twist

A delicate balance of flavors makes this winter salad a delicious, light meal to eat between breakfast and dinner while fasting.

Time: 30 minutes

Serving Size: 6 servings

Prep Time: 15 minutes

Cook Time: 15 minutes

Nutritional Facts/Info:

Calories 160

Carbs 5 g

Fat 7 g

Protein 19 g

Ingredients:

- 1 pound beef round steak
- 3 tablespoons reduced-sodium soy sauce
- 4 cups cut fresh asparagus
- 1 tablespoon rice vinegar
- 2 tablespoons sesame oil
- sesame seeds to taste
- ½ teaspoon ginger root, grated

TO SERVE

- lettuce leaves
- julienned carrot
- radishes julienned

- cilantro leaves
- a dash of lime

Directions:

1. Preheat the oven to broil.
2. On a broiler plate, position the steak.
3. Broil for approximately 6 minutes per side, or until steak is cooked as desired.
4. Remove from the oven and set aside for 5 minutes before slicing.
5. In a large saucepan bring ½ inch of water to a boil.
6. Add asparagus to the boiling water and allow to cook for 4 minutes, or until asparagus is crisp-tender.
7. Drain and set aside to cool.
8. In a separate bowl, toss the sliced beef and asparagus with soy sauce, sesame seeds, vinegar, and ginger.
9. Serve over lettuce with remaining ingredients as garnish.

Pizza Fatta Con Zucchini

Craving pizza? This zucchini base pizza eliminates the damaging carbs from your diet but keeps the traditional flavors of your favorite pizza.

Time: 45 minutes

Serving Size: 6 servings

Prep Time: 20 minutes

Cook Time: 25 minutes

Nutritional Facts/Info:

Calories 219

Carbs 10 g

Fat 12 g

Protein 14 g

Ingredients:

- 2 lightly beaten large eggs
- ½ cup mozzarella cheese, grated
- 2 cups coarsely shredded or grated zucchini (drain and squeeze dry)
- ¼ cup keto-friendly flour (almond, coconut, oat)
- ½ cup Parmesan cheese, grated
- 1 tablespoon fresh basil, minced
- 1 tablespoon olive oil
- 1 teaspoon fresh thyme, minced

TOPPINGS:

- ½ cup pepperoni, sliced
- 1 cup mozzarella cheese, grated
- 12 ounces julienned roasted sweet red peppers

Directions:

1. Preheat the oven to 450 degrees Fahrenheit

2. Combine the crust ingredients in a bowl and mix well.

3. In a 12-inch pizza pan that has been generously sprayed with cooking spray, lay your zucchini 'dough' to create a base.

4. Bake for 13-16 minutes, or until light golden brown.

5. Reduce the oven temperature to 400 degrees Fahrenheit.

6. Add your desired toppings and bake for another 10-12 minutes, or until the cheese has melted.

Garlic and Herb Roasted Chicken Thighs

Low in calories but high in filling natural proteins, this recipe is a taste of winter but can be served cool for a tasty summer lunch.

Time: 30 minutes

Serving Size: 6 servings

Prep Time: 30 minutes

Cook Time: 30 minutes

Nutritional Facts/Info:

Calories 203

Carbs 2 g

Fat 11 g

Protein 22 g

Ingredients:

- 6 boneless skinless chicken thighs
- ¼ teaspoon pepper to season
- ½ teaspoon salt to season
- 10 peeled and halved garlic cloves
- 1 tablespoon olive oil
- 1 cup chicken stock (set 2 tablespoons aside)
- ½ teaspoon fresh thyme, minced or ⅛ teaspoon dried thyme, crushed
- 1 teaspoon fresh rosemary, minced or ¼ teaspoon dried rosemary, crushed
- 1 tablespoon fresh chives, minced

Directions:

1. Season the chicken with salt and pepper before cooking.
2. Heat oil in a big cast-iron skillet over medium-high heat.
3. Add chicken to the skillet and fry on both sides until golden brown.
4. Remove pan from the heat and remove the chicken from the pan. Add garlic and brandy.
5. Return to the heat and simmer, stirring continuously, until the liquid has almost entirely evaporated (around 1-2 minutes).
6. Place the cooked chicken in the evaporated brandy sauce.
7. Add the stock, rosemary, and thyme.
8. Bring to the boil, reducing the heat to low and cook, uncovered, for 6-8 minutes or until a thermometer reads 170°.
9. Garnish with chives and serve.

Chicken Niçoise Salad

Warm southern flavors with a twist, our salad is designed to be eaten as a meal on its own.

Time: 30 minutes

Serving Size: 4 servings

Prep Time: 15 minutes

Cook Time: 15 minutes

Nutritional Facts/Info:

Calories 289

Carbs 9 g

Fat 18 g

Protein 24 g

Ingredients:

DRESSING:

- ¼ cup olive oil
- 2 tablespoons lemon juice
- 2 teaspoons lemon zest, grated
- 1 teaspoon Dijon mustard
- 2 garlic cloves, minced
- pepper to taste
- ⅛ teaspoon salt

SALAD:

- 1 5-ounce can of flaked light tuna in water, drained
- 1 teaspoon rinsed and drained capers

- 2 tablespoons pitted and sliced ripe olives
- 1 6-ounce package of ready-to-use grilled chicken breast strips, Southwest-style
- 2 cups mixed salad greens, torn or shredded
- 1 julienned medium sweet red pepper
- 1 thinly sliced small red onion
- 2 large eggs, hard-boiled and cut into wedges
- ½ pound fresh green beans, trimmed and halved, about 1 cup

Directions:

1. In a saucepan, bring water to a boil.
2. Add green beans cooking until crisp but tender.
3. Remove the beans from the pan and immerse them in ice water to cool.
4. Drain and dry with a towel.
5. In a separate mixing bowl, combine the dressing ingredients.
6. Toss tuna with olives and capers gently in a small bowl.
7. Serve on a bed of salad greens topped with the tuna green beans and the remainder of the ingredients.
8. Add salad dressing to taste.

Finger Licking Grilled Turkey With Dill

An all-time favorite cookout recipe, this tasty, tender turkey dish will have even non-keto eaters gathering around the grill.

Time: 1 hour 10 minutes

Serving Size: 6 servings

Prep Time: 10 minutes

Cook Time: 1 hour

Nutritional Facts/Info:

Calories 245

Carbs 5 g

Fat 12 g

Protein 28 g

Ingredients:

- 1 cup plain yogurt
- ⅓ cup canola oil
- ½ cup lemon juice
- ½ cup green onions, chopped
- ½ cup fresh parsley, minced
- 4 tablespoons fresh dill, minced or 4 teaspoons dill weed
- 4 minced garlic cloves
- 1 teaspoon salt to season
- teaspoon pepper to taste
- 1 teaspoon crushed dried rosemary
- 1 2.5-pound turkey breast half

Directions:

1. Preheat your oven to 350 degrees Fahrenheit.
2. Combine all ingredients except turkey in a large mixing bowl.
3. Remove half of the combined ingredients, store them in an extra-large resealable plastic bag.
4. Add the turkey breast to the resealable bag.
5. Refrigerate for 6-8 hours or overnight to marinate.
6. Cover the remaining yogurt mixture and refrigerate.
7. Once the turkey has marinated for the desired time, remove it from the marinade. Discard the marinade.
8. Place turkey in preheated oven and grill for 1 to 1 ¼ hours.
9. Baste the breast regularly with the remainder of your stored marinade.
10. Remove from the oven and let sit for 5 minutes.
11. Serve and enjoy.

Shakshuka

A classic North African dish that is rich in flavor and easy to make, Shakshuka may be traditionally eaten for breakfast but is a welcome addition to every meal.

Time: 30 minutes

Serving Size: 4 servings

Prep Time: 15 minutes

Cook Time: 15 minutes

Nutritional Facts/Info:

Calories 159

Carbs 6 g

Fat 12 g

Protein 7 g

Ingredients:

- 2 tablespoons olive oil
- 1 minced garlic clove
- 1 finely chopped medium onion
- 1 teaspoon pepper to season
- 1 teaspoon ground cumin
- 1 ½ teaspoon salt to season
- ½ to 1 teaspoon chili powder
- 2 medium roughly chopped tomatoes
- 1 teaspoon sriracha chili sauce or hot pepper sauce (optional)
- fresh cilantro, chopped
- 4 eggs, large

- toast whole pita loaves (keto-friendly)

Directions:

1. Heat the oil in a big cast-iron skillet over medium heat.
2. Add onions to the oil and cook until soft or for 4-6 minutes.
3. Add the garlic, other seasonings, and chili sauce and allow to cook for another 30 seconds.
4. Add the remainder of your vegetables and allow to stew for 4 to 6 minutes or until the mixture is thickened.
5. Create four wells in the vegetable mixture with the back of a spoon; crack an egg into each well.
6. Cook, wrapped, for an additional 4 to 6 minutes, or until egg whites are fully set and yolks are thickening but not firm.
7. Serve with pita bread and cilantro on the side.

Chapter 5: Keto Dinner Recipes

Eating a calorie-rich, healthy meal before 6 p.m. will help keep you feeling full through your fasting period at night. Should you be going into a 24 hour or 32 hour fasting period it is vitally important to ensure that you are eating a well-balanced meal that will keep your body energized through your longer fasting periods. Those who are temporarily, or full-time, on the Warrior Fasting protocol consume most of their calories between 4 and 7 p.m. and will need to incorporate most of their calorie intake during dinner.

The recipes provided in this chapter cover both calorie-rich and light meals that can be incorporated into every fasting plan. Keep in mind that dinner meals should only ever be made up of the remainder of your daily calorie intake. For example, if you have consumed 1,200 calories of a 1,400 daily calorie allowance, your dinner should only consist of 200 calories. Always be mindful of how your body is feeling, and do not participate in severely restrictive calorie fasting for periods that are longer than recommended.

Kimchi Pork Lettuce Cups

A perfectly balanced calorie meal to end your day and start your evening fast, Kimchi Pork Lettuce Cups are flavorful and filling.

Time: 20 minutes

Serving Size: 2 servings

Prep Time: 5 minutes

Cook Time: 20 minutes

Nutritional Facts/Info:

Calories 322

Carbs 6.8 g

Fat 24.3 g

Protein 19.7 g

Ingredients:

- 2 teaspoons extra virgin olive oil
- 1 finely chopped garlic clove
- 8 ounces ground pork.
- handful of fresh cilantro, chopped
- ½ cup finely chopped kimchi
- 1 teaspoon fish sauce (sugar free)
- 1½ teaspoons soy sauce
- sea salt to season
- 1 small head lettuce leaves
- lime wedges
- fresh mint

Directions:

1. In a 10-inch skillet, heat the oil over medium-high heat until it shimmers.
2. Add the garlic to the pan and sauté until it is lightly golden, or 1 to 2 minutes.
3. Add the pork, stirring lightly ensuring the pork does not crumble.
4. Reduce the heat of your pan to medium-low.
5. Combine the cilantro, kimchi, fish sauce, and soy sauce in a mixing bowl.
6. Season with salt and pepper.
7. Add the sauce combination to the pork, mixing well. Cook, stirring every couple of minutes, for another 7 to 9 minutes.
8. Arrange the lettuce leaves on a platter or large plate.
9. Carefully spoon pork over lettuce leaves.
10. Garnish with lime wedges and fresh mint. Serve immediately.

Thai Turkey Burgers

Cook on the grill, or in the oven. The rich Thai flavors of these turkey burgers will keep you full through your fasting period.

Time: 15 minutes

Serving Size: 2 servings

Prep Time: 5 minutes

Cook Time: 10 minutes

Nutritional Facts/Info:

Calories 451

Carbs 1.8 g

Fat 29 g

Protein 45.5 g

Ingredients:

- 12 ounces ground turkey
- 1 garlic clove, minced
- 1 teaspoon fresh ginger, grated
- 2 teaspoons red curry paste
- A handful cilantro stems, finely chopped
- 4 teaspoons mayonnaise
- ½ teaspoon Dijon mustard
- 2 teaspoons extra virgin olive oil
- ½ teaspoon sea salt to season
- freshly ground black pepper to season
- 2 romaine heart leaves or curly kale leaves

Directions:

1. Combine the first four ingredients in a medium mixing bowl along with half of the chopped cilantro, mixing well.
2. Roll the turkey mixture into two even balls, flattening into patties.
3. In a separate bowl, combine the mayonnaise, Dijon mustard, and the remaining cilantro.
4. Add salt and pepper to taste.
5. Heat a medium-sized skillet on medium-high.
6. Add the oil to the preheated skillet.
7. Place patties into the heated oil, cooking until the burgers are browned on the outside, around 4 or 5 minutes.
8. Flip the patties and cook for another 4 or 5 minutes, or until the other side is browned and cooked through.
9. To eat, wrap each burger in a lettuce leaf.

BBQ Flank Steak & Cabbage Slaw

The perfect cookout meal that satisfies your craving for your favorite traditional Southern summer meal.

Time: 25 minutes

Serving Size: 4 servings

Prep Time: 5 minutes

Cook Time: 20 minutes

Nutritional Facts/Info:

Calories 392

Carbs 3 g

Fat 25 g

Protein 37 g

Ingredients:

- ¼ cup ketchup, sugar-free
- 2 tablespoons melted butter
- 1 teaspoon Dijon mustard
- ½ teaspoon onion powder
- ½ teaspoon Worcestershire sauce
- ½ teaspoon freshly ground black pepper, to season
- Salt to season
- 1½ pounds flank steak
- ¼ cup mayonnaise
- 1 tablespoon apple cider vinegar
- ¼ teaspoon celery seed
- 2 cups cabbage, shredded

Directions:

1. Preheat your oven's broiler to high. Place a rack under the aluminum foil-lined broiler pan.

2. Combine the ketchup, butter, onion powder, Worcestershire sauce, and black pepper in a shallow bowl, whisking well to mix.

3. Place the steak on a plate and baste each side with the sauce.

4. Put the steak into the oven on the rack and cook for 5 to 7 minutes, or until the surface is well browned.

5. Turn the steak and cook for another 5 to 7 minutes, or until the steak is done to your taste.

6. Remove from the heat and let sit for 5 minutes. Prepare the slaw.

7. In a deep bowl, whisk together the mayonnaise, vinegar, and celery seed. Season with salt and pepper to taste.

8. Stir in the cabbage until it is thoroughly coated.

9. Refrigerate until ready to use. Can be kept in the fridge for up to a day.

10. Slice the steak, and serve with slaw.

Zoodle Beef Bolognese

Traditional Italian tastes, combined with zoodles, this meal is perfect for breaking long fasts or topping up your low daily calorie intake.

Time: 3 hours 10 minutes

Serving Size: 4 servings

Prep Time: 10 minutes

Cook Time: 3 hours

Nutritional Facts/Info:

Calories 532

Carbs 8.4 g

Fat 36.2 g

Protein 42.6 g

Ingredients:

- 4 slices chopped thick-cut bacon
- 1½ pounds ground beef
- sea salt to season
- freshly ground black pepper to season
- ¾ cup heavy cream
- 1 28-ounce can tomato purée
- zoodles pre-packaged or homemade
- Parmesan cheese, grated

Directions:

1. Place the bacon in a cool deep skillet, heating slowly to medium-high heat.

2. Once the bacon is crispy, remove it from the skillet and crumble. Season with salt and pepper to taste, and set aside.

3. Reduce the heat of your skillet to medium-low and add the ground beef to your bacon drippings. Stir often until the beef begins to crumble.

4. Add the cream and mix well, stirring occasionally.

5. Once the cream has almost evaporated, but the meat is not dry, remove it from the skillet and set it aside.

6. Add the tomato purée to your skillet, seasoning to taste.

7. Once the tomato begins to boil, reduce the heat to low, adding a few teaspoons of water to prevent sticking.

8. Return the ground beef and bacon to the skillet, turning the heat down to its lowest setting, and cook for 2 to 3 hours, stirring occasionally.

9. Bring water to boil in a pot.

10. Once the water has boiled, add your zoodles, cooking until tender.

11. Drain the zoodles well.

12. Spoon the Bolognese sauce over the zoodles. Serve immediately.

Smoky Butter Roasted Chicken

Rich in butter, calories, and flavors, our traditional Smoky Butter Roasted Chicken is the perfect Sunday lunch for the whole family.

Time: 1 hour 30 minutes

Serving Size: 4 servings

Prep Time: 20 minutes

Cook Time: 1 hour 10 minutes

Nutritional Facts/Info:

Calories 614

Carbs 0.5 g

Fat 51 g

Protein 37 g

Ingredients:

- 6 tablespoons softened butter
- 1½ teaspoons smoked paprika
- 1 grated garlic clove
- a handful chopped fresh flat-leaf parsley, chopped
- sea salt, to season
- freshly ground black pepper, to season
- 3½-pound whole chicken

Directions:

1. Preheat the oven to 450 degrees.

2. Combine the sugar, paprika, garlic, parsley, salt, and pepper in a shallow bowl.

3. Mix all spices and herbs with a fork until everything is well combined.

4. In a roasting pan, position the chicken.

5. Rub the surface of your chicken with butter.

6. Sprinkle the herbs and spices over your chicken, using your hands to evenly distribute the mixture all over the surface.

7. Cover the chicken with aluminum foil and place in the oven for 20 minutes.

8. At the 20 minute mark, pour 1/2 cup of water into the base of your roasting pan to prevent the drippings from burning and to create a natural sauce from the juices.

9. Return to the oven and roast for another 40 to 50 minutes, basting every 15 minutes.

10. The chicken is done when the juices run transparent or instant-read thermometer placed in the thigh records 165 degrees Fahrenheit.

11. Remove from the oven, let sit for 10 minutes.

12. Carve and enjoy.

Chicken Fajita Bowls

Skip the unhealthy tortillas and create a keto favorite. Rich in the zesty flavors of Mexico, this easy-to-prep meal is delicious when served over a bed of cauliflower rice.

Time: 1 hour

Serving Size: 2 servings

Prep Time: 20 minutes

Cook Time: 40 minutes

Nutritional Facts/Info:

Calories 455

Carbs 6 g

Fat 32 g

Protein 36.3 g

Ingredients:

- 2 chicken thighs
- 2 chicken legs
- 2 to 3 tablespoons softened butter
- 1 teaspoon taco seasoning (sugar free)
- sea salt, to season
- freshly ground black pepper, to season
- 1 seeded and sliced poblano pepper
- 2 chopped garlic cloves
- 1 tablespoon extra virgin olive oil
- Keto-friendly couscous
- zest of ¼ lime, zested; Reserve other quarters
- Small bunch chopped fresh cilantro

Directions:

1. Preheat the oven to 450 degrees.
2. Rub 1 to 2 tablespoons of butter over the chicken pieces.
3. Place chicken on a 9-by-13-inch rimmed baking sheet in a single layer.
4. Season with salt and pepper and a dash of taco seasoning.
5. Arrange the poblano pepper and garlic in the pan and drizzle with olive oil.
6. Cover with aluminum foil and place in the oven.
7. Roast for 15 to 20 minutes before turning the peppers to coat in the drippings.
8. If the pan seems to be too dry, add a few teaspoons of water.
9. Bake for another 15 to 20 minutes, basting the chicken with its drippings once.
10. Bring your kettle to the boil.
11. In a shallow dish, place the required amount of cauliflower couscous.
12. Fill the dish with water until couscous is submerged and cover for 15 minutes.
13. Uncover the couscous. Using a fork, fluff the mixture until light, fluffy, and breaking apart.
14. Stir in the lime zest and half of the cilantro into your couscous for a zesty flavor.

15. Divide the couscous into two broad, shallow bowls. Top with a chicken piece, the peppers, and a drizzle of the roasting pan drippings.

16. Finish with the remaining cilantro and serve!

Almond-Crusted Salmon Patties

The almonds in these easy-to-digest patties give them a wonderfully crispy texture. Flavorful and well-balanced, they're a great addition to cookouts or to freeze in larger batches for busy nights.

Time: 20 minutes

Serving Size: 4 servings

Prep Time: 5 minutes

Cook Time: 15 minutes

Nutritional Facts/Info:

Calories 369

Carbs 7 g

Fat 26 g

Protein 26 g

Ingredients:

- 2 cans, around 6 ounces wild pink salmon
- 1 tablespoon Dijon mustard
- ¼ teaspoon paprika
- a handful of chopped fresh flat-leaf parsley
- 1 large egg
- sea salt and freshly ground black pepper to season
- 1 cup almond meal
- 2 tablespoons coconut oil

Directions:

1. Place the salmon, mustard, paprika, parsley, egg, salt, pepper, as well as 1 cup almond meal to your food processor jug or bowl.
2. Pulse the ingredients until they are coarsely blended (a few chunks of salmon remaining is fine).
3. Place the salmon mixture into a deep mixing bowl, cover in plastic wrap and refrigerate for at least 1 hour.
4. Divide the salmon mixture into 8 even balls, flattening into patty shapes.
5. Use the remaining almond meal to coat each of the patties.
6. Place 1 tablespoon coconut oil into a 10-inch nonstick skillet and heat until shimmering.
7. Reduce heat to medium and place the patties in the pan, making sure not to overcrowd.
8. Cook for 3 to 4 minutes, or until patties are golden brown, then flip to cook the other side for the same amount of time.
9. Set aside to drain. Let sit for 5 minutes.
10. Serve hot.

Swedish Meatballs

High in calories, these Swedish Meatballs are easy to make and are the perfect long fast break meal.

Time: 30 minutes

Serving Size: 2 servings

Prep Time: 10 minutes

Cook Time: 20 minutes

Nutritional Facts/Info:

Calories 728

Carbs 8.4 g

Fat 51 g

Protein 59.6 g

Ingredients:

- 1 pound ground beef
- 1 egg, large
- 1 garlic clove, grated
- ¼ teaspoon fresh nutmeg, grated
- 2 tablespoons fresh flat-leaf parsley, chopped
- ¼ cup almond flour
- ½ teaspoon sea salt
- fresh ground black pepper, to season
- 2 tablespoons butter
- 1 tablespoon Dijon mustard (sugar free)
- 1 teaspoon soy sauce
- 2 teaspoons coconut flour
- ¾ cup chicken or beef broth

- ½ cup heavy cream

Directions:

1. Combine the beef, egg, garlic, nutmeg, parsley, almond flour, salt, and pepper in a large mixing bowl. Mix well, using a wooden spoon or your hands.
2. Form into eight balls, each approximately the same size.
3. Melt butter over medium heat in an 8-inch skillet.
4. Place meatballs in the skillet, making sure not to overcrowd the pan.
5. Cook for 8 to 10 minutes, rotating as desired until browned all over.
6. Place in a serving dish and set aside.
7. Reserve 1 tablespoon of the fat, discarding the remainder of the drippings.
8. Return the tablespoon of drippings to your pan, and heat to medium.
9. Stir in the mustard, soy sauce, and coconut flour over medium heat.
10. Add the broth and mix well, bringing it to a boil.
11. Reduce the heat to low and add the milk.
12. Season with salt and pepper to taste.
13. Add the meatballs back to the pan, and cook 8 to 10 minutes more until the sauce thickens.
14. Serve hot.

Magic Keto Pizza

Friday nights are pizza nights. Skip the damaging high carb crust for this quick and easy Magic Keto Pizza.

Time: 30 minutes

Serving Size: 2 to 4 servings

Prep Time: 10 minutes

Cook Time: 20 minutes

Nutritional Facts/Info:

Calories 169

Carbs 5.4 g

Fat 10 g

Protein 16 g

Ingredients:

For the crust

- 1 egg, large
- 6 ounces mozzarella cheese, grated
- 4 tablespoons softened butter
- ½ cup superfine, blanched almond flour
- 6 tablespoons coconut flour
- 2 teaspoons baking powder
- ¼ teaspoon sea salt, to season

For the pizza

- ¾ cup slow-simmered tomato sauce
- 6 ounces, mozzarella cheese, grated

- Any desired keto-friendly toppings

Directions:

1. Preheat the oven to 375 degrees.
2. In a food processor, combine the egg, mozzarella, cheese, flours, baking powder, and sea salt to create the crust.
3. Pulse until a hard ball forms.
4. Finely dust coconut flour on the counter.
5. Knead the dough for 30 to 60 seconds. If it becomes too soft, add more coconut flour to the counter to prevent it from sticking.
6. Roll the dough to ⅛-inch thick and cut into a circle if required.
7. Slide dough onto a parchment-paper-lined baking dish.
8. Lightly dust the top of the dough base with coconut flour.
9. Place in the oven and bake for 15 minutes, or until golden.
10. Remove from the oven and evenly spread with tomato sauce.
11. Add any desired keto-friendly toppings and top with the remaining mozzarella cheese.
12. Return to the oven and bake for another 15 to 20 minutes, or until the cheese is melted and bubbling and the crust is crisp.
13. Let sit for 2 minutes before slicing and serving.

Salmon Wrapped in a Parcel

This low-calorie, high nutrition meal is packed with zesty citrus flavors.

Time: 35 minutes

Serving Size: 6 servings

Prep Time: 20 minutes

Cook Time: 15 minutes

Nutritional Facts/Info:

Calories 224

Carbs 6 g

Fat 13 g

Protein 20 g

Ingredients:

- 6 slices of orange
- 6 salmon fillets, around 4 ounces each
- 6 slices of lime
- Olive oil-flavored cooking spray
- 1 pound trimmed and halved asparagus
- 1/4 teaspoon pepper to season
- 1/2 teaspoon salt to season
- 3 tablespoons lemon juice
- 2 tablespoons fresh parsley, minced

Directions:

1. Preheat the oven to 425 degrees Fahrenheit.

2. Fold six 15 x 10-inch sections of parchment or heavy-duty foil in half.

3. On one side of each piece, arrange citrus slices and place the salmon and asparagus on top.

4. Using cooking oil, lightly spray the surface of the salmon then season with salt, pepper, and parsley to taste.

5. Fold the empty side of the parchment over your ingredients and pinch the sides to create parcels.

6. Place the parcels in a shallow baking dish.

7. Bake approximately 12-15 minutes or until the salmon is pink and flakes when touched.

8. Drizzle with additional lemon juice, if desired, when serving.

Low Calorie Broiled Chicken With Parmesan Artichokes

Quick and easy to make, this recipe is low in calories and perfect for anyone who prefers a larger lunch.

Time: 15 minutes

Serving Size: 8 servings

Prep Time: 5 minutes

Cook Time: 10 minutes

Nutritional Facts/Info:

Calories 288

Carbs 4 g

Fat 21 g

Protein 22 g

Ingredients:

- 8 (approximately 2 pounds) boneless skinless chicken thighs
- 2 tablespoons olive oil
- 2 7 ½-ounce jars marinated quartered artichoke hearts, drained
- ½ teaspoon pepper, to season
- 1 teaspoon salt, to season
- 2 tablespoons fresh parsley, minced
- 1/4 cup Parmesan cheese, grated

Directions:

1. Preheat the boiler to 350 degrees Fahrenheit.

2. In a large mixing bowl, toss the chicken and artichokes with the oil, salt, and pepper.

3. Arrange the chicken and artichokes in a baking dish and cover with aluminum foil.

4. Broil 8-10 minutes, or until a thermometer inserted in the center of the chicken reads 170°. Turn chicken and artichokes halfway through cooking.

5. Once the chicken is cooked, sprinkle cheese on top and return to the oven uncovered for 1 to 2 minutes until cheese melts.

6. Serve with a parsley garnish.

Melt in Your Mouth Steak

The butter in this recipe keeps you fuller for longer, while the lean protein in the steak regenerates your muscles, making this the perfect post-workout meal.

Time: 20 minutes

Serving Size: 2 servings

Prep Time: 10 minutes

Cook Time: 10 minutes

Nutritional Facts/Info:

Calories 316

Carbs 0 g

Fat 20 g

Protein 32 g

Ingredients:

- 2 tablespoons softened butter, divided
- 1/2 teaspoon garlic, minced
- 1 teaspoon fresh parsley, minced or finely chopped
- 1 ¾-pound beef flat iron steak (can substitute for boneless top sirloin)
- 1/4 teaspoon reduced-sodium soy sauce
- 1/8 teaspoon pepper, to season
- 1/8 teaspoon salt, to season

Directions:

1. In a small mixing bowl, combine 1 tablespoon butter, parsley, garlic, and soy sauce in a mixing bowl.

2. Refrigerate mixture.

3. Season the steak with salt and pepper.

4. Place a large skillet over medium heat and melt the remaining butter in the pan.

5. Once skillet is heated, cook steak to your liking, roughly 4-7 minutes per side.

6. Remove the steak from the pan and let sit for a few minutes.

7. Remove the garlic butter from the fridge.

8. Plate steak and serve with garlic butter on the side.

Zoodles with Herby Tilapia

Quick and easy to make our herby tilapia does not compromise on its tastiness.

Time: 30 minutes

Serving Size: 4 servings

Prep Time: 15 minutes

Cook Time: 15 minutes

Nutritional Facts/Info:

Calories 203

Carbs 8 g

Fat 4 g

Protein 34 g

Ingredients:

- 1 ½ pounds zucchini (2 to 3 large)
- ¾ teaspoon salt, divided into 2 equal parts
- 1 ½ teaspoons ground cumin
- ½ teaspoon pepper
- ½ teaspoon smoked paprika
- 4, 6 ounce tilapia fillets
- ¼ tsp garlic powder
- 2 garlic cloves, minced
- 2 teaspoons olive oil
- 1 cup pico de gallo

Directions:

1. Trim ends of zucchini.
2. Using spiralizer, cut zucchini.
3. Combine the cumin, 1/2 teaspoon cinnamon, half the salt, smoked paprika, pepper, and garlic powder.
4. Sprinkle the mixed spices over the tilapia.
5. Heat the oil in a large nonstick skillet over medium-high heat.
6. Place the tilapia in batches in the pan, turning once. The fish is cooked when flakes easily with a fork, around 2-3 minutes per side.
7. Remove the fish from the pan and set it aside.
8. In the same skillet, place your zucchini and garlic over medium-high heat.
9. Toss occasionally with tongs, until slightly softened, around 1-2 minutes.
10. Season with the remaining salt.
11. Serve with tilapia and pico de gallo.

Smoky Scallops and Spinach

Smoky flavored scallops with a boost of iron-rich spinach, create a light on the stomach meal for anyone who is only looking to top up their calorie intake.

Time: 25 minutes

Serving Size: 4 servings

Prep Time: 10 minutes

Cook Time: 15 minutes

Nutritional Facts/Info:

Calories 247

Carbs 12 g

Fat 11 g

Protein 26 g

Ingredients:

- 4 pre-chopped bacon strips
- 2 finely chopped shallots
- 1 ½ pounds (around 12) sea scallops, side muscles removed
- 8 ounces, around cups fresh baby spinach
- ½ cup chicken broth, or white wine for extra smoky flavor

Directions:

1. Preheat your pan over medium heat.
2. Place bacon in the pan and cook until crisp.

3. Remove bacon from the pan and drain on paper towels.

4. Reserve 2 tablespoons of the bacon drippings and discard the rest.

5. Using paper towels, pat the scallops dry.

6. Place 1 tablespoon of the bacon drippings in your pan and heat to medium-high.

7. Place the scallops into the pan and cook for 2-3 minutes on either side or until golden brown and solid. Remove from pan.

8. With the remaining bacon drippings, cook the shallots until tender. Add wine and bring to a boil.

9. Gently add the spinach and cook until wilted.

10. Add the bacon and mix well.

11. Top with scallops and serve.

Thai Cauliflower Soup

Thai flavors permeate this amazing winter meal. Healthy and delicious, our Cauliflower Soup is a taste of Thailand without the added calories.

Time: 35 minutes

Serving Size: 10 servings

Prep Time: 10 minutes

Cook Time: 25 minutes

Nutritional Facts/Info:

Calories 111

Carbs 10 g

Fat 8 g

Protein 3 g

Ingredients:

- 2 tablespoons olive oil
- 3 tablespoons yellow curry paste
- 1 finely chopped medium onion
- 1 32-ounce carton vegetable broth (low sodium, sugar free)
- 2 medium heads cauliflower, broken into florets
- 2 tablespoons fresh cilantro, minced (optional)
- 1 cup coconut milk (no added sugar)

Directions:

1. Bring a saucepan to medium heat and add the oil.

2. Add the onion and cook, stirring until the onion is softened.

3. Add the curry powder to the onion. Stir for 1 to 2 minutes or until the curry paste is fragrant.

4. Add the cauliflower and the broth to the pot. Bring to a boil over high heat.

5. Once boiling, reduce heat to medium-low, cover and simmer for 20 minutes.

6. Add the coconut milk and stir well for one minute.

7. Remove from heat and allow to cool.

8. Puree the mixture in batches using your preferred method.

9. Reheat before eating. Garnish with fresh cilantro, if desired.

Punchy Dill Chicken

Punchy dill flavors paired with a classic chicken and broccoli dish, this meal is ideal for those who prefer a lighter dinner.

Time: 30 minutes

Serving Size: 4 servings

Prep Time: 15 minutes

Cook Time: 15 minutes

Nutritional Facts/Info:

Calories 274

Carbs 8 g

Fat 9 g

Protein 39 g

Ingredients:

- 4 6-ounce boneless skinless chicken breast, halved
- ¼ teaspoon pepper
- ½ teaspoon garlic salt
- 4 cups fresh broccoli florets
- 1 tablespoon olive oil
- 1 tablespoon keto-friendly flour
- 1 cup chicken broth
- 1 cup 2% milk
- 1 tablespoon fresh dill

Directions:

1. In a large skillet, heat the oil over medium heat.

2. Season the chicken with salt and pepper.
3. Place the chicken in the skillet and brown on both sides.
4. Remove the chicken from the pan and set it aside.
5. In the same skillet, add broccoli and broth. Bring to a boil.
6. Reduce heat to low, cover, and cook for 3-5 minutes, or until broccoli is tender.
7. Remove the broccoli from the pan, with a slotted spoon, reserving the broth.
8. Mix flour, dill, and milk in a small bowl until smooth.
9. Stir the flour mixture into the broth.
10. Bring to a boil, stirring constantly for 1-2 minutes or until thickened.
11. Add the chicken to the skillet and cook, covered, over medium heat.
12. Serve with broccoli on the side.

Steak and Eggs With a Warm Summer Salad

A healthy variation to your traditional steak, egg, and fries. Replace the fries with your favorite Keto vegetable.

Time: 30 minutes

Serving Size: 4 servings

Prep Time: 15 minutes

Cook Time: 15 minutes

Nutritional Facts/Info:

Calories 344

Carbs 7 g

Fat 21 g

Protein 33 g

Ingredients:

- 1 1-pound beef skirt steak (can be substituted with flank steak))
- 2 tablespoons butter, divided equally
- 1 teaspoon Montreal keto-friendly steak seasoning (no sugar added)
- 1 medium yellow summer squash, cut into ¼-inch slices
- 1 medium zucchini, cut into ¼-inch slices
- 6 cups fresh baby spinach
- 1 medium chopped sweet red pepper
- ¼ teaspoon pepper, to season
- ½ teaspoon salt, to season
- ¼ cup Parmesan cheese, grated
- 4 eggs, large

Directions:

1. Season the steak with salt and pepper.
2. Heat a large skillet over medium heat.
3. Place the steak into the pan and cook for 3-5 minutes on either side or until the steak is done to your preference.
4. Remove the steak from the pan. Let stand for 5 minutes.
5. In the same skillet, melt 1 tablespoon of butter.
6. Add the zucchini, squash, and red pepper, cooking for 5-7 minutes, until the vegetables are tender-crisp.
7. Add the spinach, salt, and pepper. Cook and stir for an additional 2 minutes or until spinach is wilted.
8. Plate vegetables and return the pan to the stove.
9. Heat the remaining butter.
10. Crack the eggs into the pan and fry according to desired doneness.
11. Plate your steak, eggs, on the vegetables. Top with grated Parmesan.
12. Serve and enjoy.

Spicy Mexican Cabbage and Green Chili Soup

A hearty, spicy soup that is low in calories, and rich in flavor.

Time: 30 minutes

Serving Size: 6 servings

Prep Time: 15 minutes

Cook Time: 15 minutes

Nutritional Facts/Info:

Calories 186

Carbs 10 g

Fat 9 g

Protein 17 g

Ingredients:

- 1 pound lean ground beef
- ¾ teaspoon garlic powder
- ½ teaspoon salt, to season
- 1 tablespoon olive oil
- ¼ teaspoon pepper, to season
- 6 cups cabbage, roughly chopped
- 1 medium chopped onion
- 2 cups water
- 3 4-ounce can green chiles, finely chopped
- 2 tablespoons fresh cilantro, minced
- 1 14 ½-ounce can beef broth (reduced sodium)
- Optional toppings: pico de gallo and reduced-fat sour cream

Directions:

1. Using a large saucepan, cook beef over medium-high heat. Stir frequently, using a wooden spoon or spatula to break up any clumps. Cook until no pink remains, approximately 7 minutes.
2. Add your seasoning and stir well.
3. Remove the meat from the pan and set it aside.
4. In the same pan, heat the oil.
5. Add the onion and cabbage and cook on medium heat until tender, approximately 6 minutes.
6. Add the beef, chilis, water, and broth, bringing to the boil.
7. Once boiling, reduce heat to low, cover for 10 minutes to allow flavors to mix.
8. Add the cilantro and mix well.
9. Serve topped with pico de gallo and sour cream.

Classic BLT With a Twist

The classic BLT with a twist, this salad can be eaten as a side dish or as a main meal.

Time: 20 minutes

Serving Size: 8 servings

Prep Time: 10 minutes

Cook Time: 10 minutes

Nutritional Facts/Info:

Calories 281

Carbs 5 g

Fat 19 g

Protein 23 g

Ingredients:

- ½ cup keto-friendly mayonnaise
- 2 tablespoons onion, finely chopped
- 3 to 4 tablespoons barbecue sauce (no added sugar)
- ¼ teaspoon pepper, to season
- 1 tablespoon lemon juice
- 2 large tomatoes, chopped
- 8 cups salad greens, torn or shredded
- 10 pre-cooked bacon strips, diced or crumbled
- 1 ½ pounds pre-cooked boneless, skinless chicken breasts, shredded or sliced
- 2 sliced hard-boiled eggs, large

Directions:

1. To make dressing, combine the first 5 ingredients in a deep mixing bowl. Stir well.

2. Cover and chill in the refrigerator.

3. In a separate bowl, combine the salad greens, tomatoes, onions, chicken, and bacon.

4. Top with eggs and dressing.

Grecian Ribeye Steaks

Classic Grecian flavors combined with a steak that is grilled to perfection, this meal is balanced in nutrition and calories, and quick to prepare.

Time: 30 minutes

Serving Size: 4 servings

Prep Time: 15 minutes

Cook Time: 15 minutes

Nutritional Facts/Info:

Calories 597

Carbs 11 g

Fat 44 g

Protein 37 g

Ingredients:

- 4 chopped plum tomatoes
- ⅔ cup Greek olives, pitted
- 1 cup red onion, chopped
- ¼ cup lemon juice, divided in half
- 1/4 cup fresh cilantro, minced
- 2 minced garlic cloves
- 2 tablespoons olive oil
- 1 cup feta cheese, crumbled
- 2 ¾-pound beef ribeye steaks

Directions:

1. Combine 2 tbsp lemon juice, 1 tablespoon of olive oil, tomatoes, onion, olives, cilantro, and garlic in a bowl. Mix well to make relish.

2. Cover and refrigerate.

3. Season your steak and drizzle with the last of the lemon juice.

4. Heat a non-stick pan over medium heat. Place your steak in the pan and fry for 5-7 minutes on either side until done.

5. Remove steak from the pan. Let sit for 5 minutes.

6. Service with feta crumbled on top and relish on the side.

Chapter 6: Keto Snack Recipes

While snacking should be avoided under normal circumstances, Intermittent fasting encourages eating during your eating windows as long as you remain within your set calorie intake. Sometimes snacking is unavoidable! Strenuous workouts and sugar dips can have you reaching for unhealthy substitutes. Rather than diving for the crisps, stick to hunger satiating good fats and snacks that help to balance sugar and energy levels. Try to avoid zero-calorie drinks, like coffee, that stimulate your appetite opting for Keto-friendly snacks.

Be mindful of zero-calorie drinks that make you hungry, and try to avoid these when snacking. Also, when snackish, take the time to consider whether you are actually hungry or whether you are confusing thirst for hunger. The only rules you should follow when snacking with intermittent fasting are; never eat over your prescribed calorie intake, and do not eat after 6 p.m. or 7 p.m., depending on your sleep and wake cycles.

Smoky Cheese Dip

Time: 2 hours 15 minutes

Serving Size: 4 servings

Prep Time: 15 minutes

Cook Time: 2 hours

Nutritional Facts/Info:

Calories 261

Carbs 3 g

Fat 23 g

Protein 11 g

Ingredients:

- 2 8-ounce packages cream cheese, cubed
- 1 cup half-and-half cream
- 1 teaspoon prepared mustard
- 4 cups cheddar cheese, grated
- 1 teaspoon dried onion, crushed
- 2 teaspoons Worcestershire sauce
- 16 pre-cooked bacon strips, diced or crumbled
- Tortilla chips or toasted French bread slices (keto-friendly)

Directions:

1. Combine the cream cheese, cream, mustard, cheese, onion and Worcestershire sauce in a 1-1/2-quart slow cooker.

2. Cover, cook on low and stir regularly for 2-3 hours until cheeses are melted.

3. Stir in the bacon just before serving.

4. Serve with warm keto tortilla chips or toasted keto bread.

Italian Antipasto Cheese Ring

Time: 25 minutes

Serving Size: 16 servings

Prep Time: 25 minutes

Cook Time: 0 minutes

Nutritional Facts/Info:

Calories 168

Carbs 2 g

Fat 16 g

Protein 6 g

Ingredients:

- 1 8-ounce package cream cheese, cold
- ⅓ cup pimiento-stuffed olives
- 1 10-ounce package sharp white cheddar cheese
- ¼ cup balsamic vinegar
- ⅓ cup Greek olives, pitted
- 1 tablespoon fresh parsley, minced
- ¼ cup olive oil
- 2 garlic cloves, minced
- 1 tablespoon fresh basil, minced or 1 teaspoon dried basil, crushed
- Toasted French bread baguette slices
- 1 2-ounce jar pimiento strips, drained and chopped

Directions:

1. Slice cream cheese in half lengthwise. Then, cut each half into 1/4-inch slices.

2. Repeat with white cheddar cheese.

3. Arrange the cheeses in a circle on a serving tray, alternating cheddar and cream cheese strips.

4. Place both types of olives in the middle of the serving tray.

5. Whisk together the oil, parsley, basil, vinegar, and garlic in a shallow bowl. Drizzle the mixture over the arranged platter.

6. Sprinkle pimientos on top.

7. Cover and refrigerate for a minimum of 8 hours or overnight.

8. Serve with slices of keto baguette.

French Tapenade With Red Peppers and Almonds

Time: 15 minutes

Serving Size: 2 servings

Prep Time: 15 minutes

Cook Time: 0 minutes

Nutritional Facts/Info:

Calories 58

Carbs 3 g

Fat 4 g

Protein 1 g

Ingredients:

- 3 peeled garlic cloves
- ½ cup almonds, blanched
- 2 cups sweet red peppers, roasted
- 2 tablespoons olive oil
- ⅓ cup tomato paste
- ¼ teaspoon pepper, to season
- ¼ teaspoon salt, to season
- Keto-friendly toasted French bread baguette slices
- fresh basil, minced

Directions:

1. Bring 2 cups of water to a boil in a small saucepan.

2. Place the garlic in the boiling water and cook, uncovered, for 6-8 minutes or until garlic is tender.

3. Drain the water and pat the garlic dry.

4. In a food processor, combine red peppers, almonds, tomato paste, oil, garlic, salt, and pepper; pulse until smooth.

5. Place in a small bowl and refrigerate for 4 hours.

6. Garnish with basil leaves.

7. Serve with slices of keto baguette.

Chicken-Cheese Skewers

Time: 20 minutes

Serving Size: 8 servings

Prep Time: 20 minutes

Cook Time: 0 minutes

Nutritional Facts/Info:

Calories 93

Carbs 3 g

Fat 4 g

Protein 12 g

Ingredients:

- ½ teaspoon salt, to season
- ⅛ teaspoon pepper, to season
- ½ teaspoon chili powder
- ½ cup balsamic vinegar
- ½ pound cubed, boneless skinless chicken breast
- 5 ounces mozzarella cheese, cubed
- 2 teaspoons olive oil
- 16 cherry or grape tomatoes

Directions:

1. In a large mixing bowl, combine chicken cubes and vinegar with a mixture of salt, chili powder, and pepper.
2. Toss the chicken until coated and cover the bowl with plastic wrap.

3. Refrigerate for 3-4 hours.

4. Drain the chicken and dispose of the marinade.

5. In a large skillet, add the chicken and cook over medium heat. The chicken is cooked once the flesh is white and juices are clear.

6. Remove cooked chicken from the heat and set aside to cool.

7. Thread chicken, cheese, and tomatoes onto wooden skewers in random order.

8. Serve cold.

Pimiento and Cheese Deviled Eggs

Time: 15 minutes

Serving Size: 12 servings

Prep Time: 15 minutes

Cook Time: 0 minutes

Nutritional Facts/Info:

Calories 67

Carbs 1 g

Fat 5 g

Protein 4 g

Ingredients:

- 6 hard-boiled eggs, large
- 2 tablespoons mayonnaise
- ¼ cup sharp cheddar cheese, finely grated
- 2 teaspoons sweet onion, finely chopped
- 4 teaspoons pimientos, drained and diced
- 1 small minced garlic clove
- 1 teaspoon Dijon mustard
- ⅛ teaspoon pepper, to season
- ¼ teaspoon salt, to season

GARNISHING

- pimiento, diced
- sharp cheddar cheese, finely grated

Directions:

1. Cut eggs in half lengthwise.
2. Separate the egg yolks from whites. Place yolks in a separate bowl, and keep the whites.
3. Mash the yolks in a mixing bowl.
4. Add pimientos, onion, cheese, mayonnaise, garlic, salt, mustard, and pepper to the mashed yolk.
5. Place the mixture in a piping bag.
6. Pipe the egg yolk mixture into the center of your egg whites.
7. Cover and refrigerate until serving.
8. Garnish with a sprinkling of pimientos and cheese.

Smoky Salmon Cream Cheese Dip

Time: 15 minutes

Serving Size: 2 ½ cups

Prep Time: 15 minutes

Cook Time: 0 minutes

Nutritional Facts/Info:

Calories 96

Carbs 1 g

Fat 9 g

Protein 3 g

Ingredients:

- 2 8-ounce packages softened cream cheese
- 1 tablespoon Worcestershire sauce
- 1 4-ounce package smoked salmon
- 1 tablespoon lemon juice
- ¼ teaspoon coarsely ground pepper, to season
- 3 tablespoons horseradish sauce
- ¼ teaspoon Creole seasoning
- walnuts, chopped
- fresh dill, snipped
- assorted keto crackers

Directions:

1. In a food processor, combine the cream cheese, Worcestershire, salmon, lemon juice, pepper,

horseradish, and Creole seasoning and process until smooth.

2. Form into a ball and refrigerate before serving.

3. Place on a serving platter and top with walnuts and dill.

4. Serve with keto crackers on the side.

Sweet Red Pepper Seasoned Cheese

Time: 30 minutes

Serving Size: 2 cups

Prep Time: 30 minutes

Cook Time: 0 minutes

Nutritional Facts/Info:

Calories 121

Carbs 1 g

Fat 11 g

Protein 5 g

Ingredients:

- 2 8-ounce blocks white cheddar cheese
- ¾ cup roasted sweet red peppers, coarsely chopped
- 2 8-ounce packages cream cheese
- ¼ cup white wine vinegar
- ½ cup olive oil
- 3 tablespoons green onions, chopped
- ¼ cup balsamic vinegar
- 2 tablespoons fresh basil, minced
- 3 tablespoons fresh parsley, minced
- 3 garlic cloves, minced
- 1 tablespoon sugar
- ½ teaspoon pepper
- ½ teaspoon salt
- Keto-friendly toasted sliced French bread

Directions:

1. Each block of cheddar cheese should be cut into twenty 1/4-inch slices.

2. Each block of cream cheese should be cut into 18 slices.

3. For each stack, sandwich 9 cream cheese slices between 10 cheddar slices.

4. Fill a 13x9-inch baking dish with the stacks.

5. Combine the roasted peppers, vinegars, oil, onions, basil, parsley, garlic, sugar, salt, and pepper in a small bowl and mix to combine.

6. Drizzle the vegetable mixture over the cheese stacks.

7. Cover and chill the cheese blocks overnight, turning them once.

8. Drain the leftover marinade before serving.

9. Serve with keto crackers or toasted keto bread.

Italian Style Portobello Mushrooms

Time: 20 minutes

Serving Size: 4 servings

Prep Time: 20 minutes

Cook Time: 0 minutes

Nutritional Facts/Info:

Calories 273

Carbs 9 g

Fat 22 g

Protein 9 g

Ingredients:

- 4 4-½-inch, large portobello mushroom
- 1 minced garlic clove
- 2 tablespoons olive oil
- 4 ounces feta cheese, crumbled
- ¼ teaspoon salt, to season
- ½ cup prepared pesto (no added sugar)

Directions:

1. Remove stems from the mushrooms. Remove gills from mushroom caps with a spoon.

2. Combine oil and garlic in a shallow bowl; brush over mushrooms.

3. Season with salt.

4. Combine the cheese and pesto in a shallow dish.

5. Place the mushrooms on a greased heavy-duty foil sheet (about 12-in. square).

6. Cover the mushrooms in foil. Grill, stem side up, over medium heat for 8-10 minutes. Mushrooms are cooked when they become soft.

7. Spread the cheese mixture over the mushrooms, cover and grill for 2-3 minutes.

Summer Fresh Chicken Dip

Time: 30 minutes

Serving Size: 36 servings

Prep Time: 30 minutes

Cook Time: 0 minutes

Nutritional Facts/Info:

Calories 97

Carbs 4 g

Fat 6 g

Protein 7 g

Ingredients:

- 2 tablespoons reduced-sodium soy sauce
- 2 minced garlic cloves
- 4 teaspoons sesame oil
- 3 8-ounce packages cream cheese (reduced-fat if you prefer)
- 4 cups pre-cooked chicken breast, shredded
- 2 cups fresh baby spinach, chopped
- 1 10-ounce jar sweet-and-sour sauce (no added sugar)
- ½ cup chopped salted peanuts
- 1 cup sliced green onions, thinly sliced
- Keto-friendly crackers

Directions:

1. In a large bowl, toss chicken with soy sauce, sesame oil, and garlic.

2. Cover and refrigerate for at least 1 hour.

3. To serve, scoop a generous portion of chicken onto a bed of spinach. Add cream cheese on the side, and drizzle with sweet-and-sour sauce.

4. Garnish with green onions and peanuts.

5. Cover and chill for 2 hours minimum. Then serve with keto crackers on the side.

Cheese and Chives Ball

Time: 15 minutes

Serving Size: 2 cups

Prep Time: 15 minutes

Cook Time: 0 minutes

Nutritional Facts/Info:

Calories 145

Carbs 2 g

Fat 14 g

Protein 3 g

Ingredients:

- 1 8-ounce package cream cheese, softened
- ¼ cup softened butter
- 1 cup blue cheese, crumbled
- 1 tablespoon chives, finely chopped
- 1 4-¼-ounce can ripe olives, pitted and chopped
- Keto-friendly crackers
- ¾ cup walnuts, chopped

Directions:

1. In a large mixing bowl, combine the cream cheese and blue cheese, mixing until a creamy consistency is achieved.//
2. Add the olives and chives and mix well.
3. Cover and refrigerate for at least 1 hour.

4. Using your hands, mold the cheese mixture into the shape of a ball, then roll it in walnuts.

5. Wrap and refrigerate for another 1 hour.

6. Serve with keto crackers on the side.

Creamy Parmesan Caulimash

Time: 30 minutes

Serving Size: 6 servings

Prep Time: 30 minutes

Cook Time: 0 minutes

Nutritional Facts/Info:

Calories 154

Carbs 8 g

Fat 11 g

Protein 8 g

Ingredients:

- 2 ½ pounds cauliflower (about 1 large cauliflower), broken into florets
- ⅓ cup heavy whipping cream or half-and-half cream
- 1 cup Parmesan cheese, grated and divided
- ½ teaspoon pepper
- 1 tablespoon butter (unsalted)
- fresh parsley, minced (optional)

Directions:

1. In a big saucepan, combine 1 inch of water and the cauliflower.

2. Using high heat, bring water to a boil. Cover and cook for approximately 10 minutes or until the cauliflower is tender.

3. Drain the water.

4. Mash the cauliflower to its desired consistency.

5. In a separate bowl, combine cream, 1/2 cup cheese, pepper and butter.

6. Add this mixture to your hot cauliflower mash and mix well.

7. Before serving, top with the remaining cheese and parsley, if desired

Sausage Stuffed Mushrooms Caps

Time: 35 minutes

Serving Size: 12 servings

Prep Time: 15 minutes

Cook Time: 20 minutes

Nutritional Facts/Info:

Calories 59

Carbs 2 g

Fat 5 g

Protein 2 g

Ingredients:

- 12 large mushrooms, fresh
- 2 tablespoons onion, chopped
- 2 tablespoons butter, divided into 2 equal parts
- ¼ teaspoon dried basil, crushed
- 1 tablespoon lemon juice
- 4 ounces Italian sausage
- salt and pepper, to season
- 2 tablespoons bread crumbs, dried
- 1 tablespoon fresh parsley, chopped
- green onions, thinly sliced (optional)
- 2 tablespoons Parmesan cheese, grated

Directions:

1. Remove mushroom stems and place caps in a greased 15x10x1-inch baking pan.

2. Finely chop the stems. Loosely wrap with paper towels then squeeze to remove the extra moisture.

3. Preheat the oven to 400 degrees Fahrenheit.

4. Over medium heat, use a large skillet to heat butter until it melts.

5. Add the onion and mushroom stems to the pan and cook until tender.

6. Add lemon juice to the pan and cook until the lemon juice has almost completely evaporated. Allow to cool slightly.

7. Combine the bacon, parsley, and onion mixture in a mixing bowl and spoon into mushroom caps.

8. Sprinkle the top of your mushroom caps with bread crumbs and cheese.

9. Dot the remaining butter on top.

10. Bake for 15-20 minutes, basting regularly with pan juices until sausage is cooked through.

11. Garnish with green onions.

Cream Cheese and Pork Stuffed Jalapenos

Time: 35 minutes

Serving Size: 44 servings

Prep Time: 20 minutes

Cook Time: 15 minutes

Nutritional Facts/Info:

Calories 56

Carbs 1 g

Fat 5 g

Protein 2 g

Ingredients:

- 1 pound pork sausage
- 1 cup Parmesan cheese, grated
- 1 8-ounce package softened cream cheese
- Ranch salad dressing (optional)
- 22 large halved, seeded jalapeno peppers

Directions:

1. Preheat your oven to 425 degrees Fahrenheit
2. Heat a large skillet over medium heat.
3. Add the sausage to the skillet and cook until it is no longer pink. Set aside to cool.
4. Remove sausage casing and crumble the meat.

5. Combine the cream cheese and Parmesan cheese in a shallow mixing bowl. Fold in the sausage meat.

6. Fill each half of a jalapeno with about 1 tablespoon of the mixture.

7. Place the jalapenos in two 13x9-inch ungreased baking dishes.

8. Bake uncovered for 15-20 minutes or until the filling is slightly browned and bubbly.

9. If desired, drizzle with ranch dressing.

Asparagus in a Blanket

Time: 30 minutes

Serving Size: 2 servings

Prep Time: 30 minutes

Cook Time: 4 to 6 minutes

Nutritional Facts/Info:

Calories 120

Carbs 4 g

Fat 8 g

Protein 9 g

Ingredients:

- 10 trimmed fresh asparagus spears
- ⅛ teaspoon pepper, to season
- Cooking spray
- 5 bacon strips

Directions:

1. Arrange asparagus on waxed paper and cover with cooking spray.
2. Season with pepper and toss to coat.
3. Half bacon strips.
4. Wrap a strip of bacon around each spear and secure with toothpicks at the ends.

5. Heat a pan on medium heat and place bacon-wrapped spears in the pain.

6. Cook for 4-6 minutes on each side or until the bacon is crisp.

7. Remove toothpicks and serve.

Garlic and Parmesan Spinach Bake

Time: 25 minutes

Serving Size: 6 servings

Prep Time: 25 minutes

Cook Time: 0 minutes

Nutritional Facts/Info:

Calories 239

Carbs 7 g

Fat 21 g

Protein 10 g

Ingredients:

- 2 pounds baby spinach, fresh
- 5 tablespoons butter
- 1 tablespoon Italian seasoning
- 3 minced garlic cloves
- 1 cup Parmesan cheese, grated
- ¾ teaspoon salt, to season

Directions:

1. Preheat the oven to 400 degrees Fahrenheit.
2. Bring 5 cups of water to a boil in a stockpot.
3. Cook spinach, for 1 minute or until spinach is wilted.
4. Drain thoroughly.

5. Melt butter in a small skillet over medium-low heat.

6. Add the garlic, Italian seasoning, and salt to the pan, cooking until the garlic is soft, around 1-2 minutes.

7. In a greased 8-in. square baking dish, spread the wilted spinach.

8. Drizzle with the butter mixture and finish with the cheese.

9. Bake for 10-15 minutes, uncovered, until the cheese begins to brown.

Pigs in a Jalapeno Blanket

Time: 25 minutes

Serving Size: 24 minutes

Prep Time: 25 minutes

Cook Time: 0 minutes

Nutritional Facts/Info:

Calories 97

Carbs 1 g

Fat 9 g

Protein 3 g

Ingredients:

- 24 jalapeno peppers, fresh
- 12 halved bacon strips
- ¾ pound pork sausage

Directions:

1. Wash peppers and slit down the middle.
2. Remove the seeds from the peppers and discard them.
3. Cook sausages over medium heat until they are longer pink inside.
4. Stuff peppers with sausage and wrap in bacon, securing with toothpicks.

5. Grill peppers over medium heat, turning regularly until peppers are tender and bacon is crisp, around 15 minutes.

Piacenza Asparagus

Time: 35 minutes

Serving Size: 8 servings

Prep Time: 20 minutes

Cook Time: 15 minutes

Nutritional Facts/Info:

Calories 95

Carbs 4 g

Fat 8 g

Protein 3 g

Ingredients:

- 1 ½ pounds fresh asparagus, tailed
- 3 tablespoons pine nuts, roughly chopped
- 1 ½ cups halved baby tomatoes (grape or cherry variety)
- 2 minced garlic cloves
- 3 tablespoons olive oil, divided into 3 equal parts
- ½ teaspoon pepper, to season
- 1 teaspoon, salt, to season
- ⅓ cup Parmesan cheese, grated
- 1 tablespoon lemon juice
- 1 teaspoon lemon zest

Directions:

1. Preheat the oven to 400 degrees Fahrenheit.

2. In a foil-lined 15x10x1-in. baking pan, arrange the asparagus, tomatoes, and pine nuts.
3. Place garlic, salt, pepper, and 2 tablespoons of oil in a mixing bowl, whisking to combine.
4. Drizzle over asparagus and toss to coat.
5. Cook for 15-20 minutes until the asparagus is tender.
6. Drizzle the remaining oil and lemon juice over the top, then top with the cheese and lemon zest.
7. Give one final toss before serving.

Cheesy Portobello Mushrooms

Time: 30 minutes

Serving Size: 6 servings

Prep Time: 30 minutes

Cook Time: 0 minutes

Nutritional Facts/Info:

Calories 201

Carbs 9 g

Fat 13 g

Protein 12 g

Ingredients:

- ¾ cup ricotta cheese (reduced fat if preferred)
- ½ cup shredded mozzarella cheese
- ¾ cup Parmesan cheese, grated and divided into equal parts
- ⅛ teaspoon pepper, to season
- 2 tablespoons fresh parsley, minced
- 1 large tomato, cut into 6 slices
- 6 portobello mushrooms, large
- 3 tablespoons almonds or pine nuts, toasted, and roughly diced
- ¾ cup basil leaves, fresh
- 2 tablespoons olive oil
- 1 small garlic clove
- 2 to 3 teaspoons water

Directions:

1. Mix ricotta cheese, 1/4 cup Parmesan cheese, mozzarella cheese, parsley, and pepper in a bowl. Set aside.

2. Remove stems from mushrooms. Scrape and remove gills with a spoon. Discard stems.

3. Fill the mushroom caps halfway with the ricotta mixture.

4. Heat a skillet to medium heat and dry fry the mushroom caps for 8-10 minutes, or until mushrooms are soft.

5. In a food processor, pulse basil, almonds, and garlic until finely chopped.

6. Pulse in the remaining Parmesan cheese.

7. Gradually add enough oil and water to achieve the desired consistency.

8. Before serving, drizzle the sauce over the stuffed mushrooms.

Roquefort Jumbo Shrimp

Time: 20 minutes

Serving Size: 24 servings

Prep Time: 20 minutes

Cook Time: 0 minutes

Nutritional Facts/Info:

Calories 43

Carbs 0 g

Fat 2 g

Protein 6 g

Ingredients:

- 3 ounces softened cream cheese
- ¼ cup blue cheese, crumbled
- ⅔ cup fresh parsley, minced and divided into equal parts
- ½ teaspoon Creole mustard
- 1 teaspoon shallot, finely chopped
- 24 peeled, deveined, and cooked jumbo shrimp

Directions:

1. Beat the cream cheese in a small mixing bowl until a smooth consistency is achieved.

2. Combine 1/3 cup parsley, blue cheese, shallot, and mustard in a mixing bowl.

3. Fold in the cream cheese, mixing well.

4. Cover the bowl and refrigerate for at least 1 hour before serving.

5. Make a deep slit down the back of each shrimp, stopping between 1/4 to 1/2 inch from the bottom.

6. Fill with cream cheese mixture and remaining parsley, pressing the mixture into the flesh.

Spicy Pecan Cheese Spread

Time: 20 minutes

Serving Size: 2 cups

Prep Time: 15 minutes

Cook Time: 5 minutes

Nutritional Facts/Info:

Calories 139

Carbs 6 g

Fat 12 g

Protein 3 g

Ingredients:

- 1 8-ounce package softened cream cheese
- 1 cup pecan nuts, finely chopped
- 1 cup sharp white cheddar cheese, grated
- ¼ cup jalapeno pepper jelly
- 4 finely chopped green onions
- keto-friendly crackers

Directions:

1. Mix together cream cheese, cheddar cheese, pecans, and green onions in a mixing bowl until smooth.

2. Shape the cheese mixture into the desired shape on a baking tray, covering with plastic wrap.

3. Refrigerate for at least 2 hours.

4. Can be served with warm jelly (heat in the microwave) or cold.

Italian-Style Artichoke Hearts

Time: 15 minutes

Serving Size: 12 servings

Prep Time: 15 minutes

Cook Time: 0 minutes

Nutritional Facts/Info:

Calories 192

Carbs 5 g

Fat 16 g

Protein 7 g

Ingredients:

- 2 7-½-ounce jars artichoke hearts, marinated type
- 2 tablespoons olive oil
- 2 tablespoons red wine vinegar
- 1 pound sliced fresh mozzarella
- 6 sliced plum or cherry tomatoes
- Coarsely ground pepper, to season
- 2 cups fresh basil leaves, loosely packed

Directions:

1. Drain the artichokes and set aside 1/2 cup of the brine.

2. Whisk together the vinegar, oil, and reserved brine in a small bowl.

3. Arrange the artichokes, onions, mozzarella cheese, and basil on a serving platter.

4. Drizzle with vinegar mixture.

5. Season with coarsely ground pepper

Texan Poppers with Spicy Sausage Dip

Time: 3 hours 15 minutes

Serving Size: 24 servings

Prep Time: 15 minutes

Cook Time: 3 hours

Nutritional Facts/Info:

Calories 180

Carbs 2 g

Fat 15 g

Protein 8 g

Ingredients:

- 1 pound pork sausage, spicy
- 12 ounces (about 4 cups) Parmesan cheese, shredded
- 2 8-ounce packages cream cheese, cubed
- 1 4-ounce can green chiles, chopped undrained
- 1 cup sour cream
- assorted fresh vegetables

Directions:

1. Cook sausage in a large skillet over medium heat for 6-8 minutes or until no longer pink. Set aside to cool.
2. Remove sausage casings and crumble sausage contents.
3. Place the sausage crumbles into a 3-quart slow cooker.

4. Combine cream cheese, Parmesan cheese, sour cream, chilies, and peppers in the slow cooker.

5. Cook, covered, on low for 3-3 1/2 hours or until cooked through.

6. Stir well before serving. Serve with vegetables on the side.

Zesty Broccoli Roast

Time: 25 minutes

Serving Size: 8 servings

Prep Time: 25 minutes

Cook Time: 0 minutes

Nutritional Facts/Info:

Calories 84

Carbs 7 g

Fat 6 g

Protein 4 g

Ingredients:

- 1 ½ pounds fresh broccoli florets
- ½ teaspoon lemon juice
- 2 tablespoons olive oil
- ¼ teaspoon coarsely ground pepper, to season
- 1/4 teaspoon salt, to season
- 2 teaspoons fresh lemon zest, grated
- ¼ cup almonds, coarsely chopped

Directions:

1. Preheat the oven to 450 degrees Fahrenheit.
2. In a big mixing bowl, toss the broccoli with the lemon juice, oil, 1/8 teaspoon pepper and salt until well mixed.
3. Fill a 15x10x1 inch baking pan halfway with the vegetables.

4. Roast for 10-15 minutes, or until the vegetables are tender.

5. Toss in the remaining pepper, the almonds, and the lemon zest to serve.

Spinach and Cheese Marinara Dip

Time: 2 hours 20 minutes

Serving Size: 16 servings

Prep Time: 20 minutes

Cook Time: 2 hours

Nutritional Facts/Info:

Calories 197

Carbs 4 g

Fat 16 g

Protein 9 g

Ingredients:

- 1 12-ounce jar roasted sweet red peppers
- 1 10-ounce package frozen spinach, chopped, thawed and squeezed dry
- 1 6-½-ounce jar quartered artichoke hearts, marinated
- 1 ½ cups Asiago cheese, grated
- 8 ounces fresh mozzarella cheese, grated
- 1 cup feta cheese, crumbled
- 6 ounces softened cream cheese
- ⅓ cup fresh basil, minced
- ⅓ cup Provolone cheese, grated
- 2 tablespoons mayonnaise
- ¼ cup red onion, finely chopped
- 2 garlic cloves, minced
- keto-friendly crackers

Directions:

1. Drain and chop peppers and artichokes, reserving 2 tablespoons of liquid from each.

2. Combine spinach, cheeses, basil, mayonnaise, onion, garlic, artichoke hearts, and peppers in a 3-quart slow cooker sprayed with cooking spray.

3. Combine the reserved pepper and artichoke liquids in a mixing bowl giving it a light stir.

4. Add the liquid to the slow cooker.

5. Cook for 2 hours on high. Do not break the seal.

6. After 2 hours, stir and cook for another 30-60 minutes, or until the cheese is melted.

7. Stir before eating and serve with crackers.

Black and White Truffles

Time: 25 minutes

Serving Size: 36 servings

Prep Time: 25 minutes

Cook Time: 0 minutes

Nutritional Facts/Info:

Calories 80

Carbs 3 g

Fat 7 g

Protein 3 g

Ingredients:

- 2 4-ounce logs fresh goat cheese
- 6 tablespoons Parmesan cheese, grated
- 1 8-ounce carton Mascarpone cheese
- 1 ½ teaspoons olive oil
- 3 minced garlic cloves
- ¾ teaspoon fresh lemon zest, grated
- 1 ½ teaspoons white balsamic vinegar
- 3 ounces dried figs, chopped
- 3 ounces Prosciutto, chopped
- ¼ teaspoon pepper, to season
- 3 tablespoons fresh parsley, minced
- 1 cup pine nuts, toasted and chopped

Directions:

1. Combine all ingredients, except pine nuts in a mixing bowl and stir until well mixed.

2. Form 36 balls from the above ingredients.

3. Roll the balls in pine nuts and refrigerate to set.

Waist-Friendly Chocolate Cups

Time: 18 minutes

Serving Size: 12 servings

Prep Time: 15 minutes

Cook Time: 3 minutes

Nutritional Facts/Info:

Calories 246

Carbs 3.3 g

Fat 26 g

Protein 3.4 g

Ingredients:

- 1 cup coconut oil
- 2 tablespoons heavy cream
- ½ cup natural peanut butter
- 1 teaspoon liquid stevia
- 1 tablespoon cocoa powder
- ¼ teaspoon salt
- ¼ teaspoon vanilla extract
- 1 ounce roasted salted peanuts, chopped

Directions:

1. In a saucepan over low heat, melt coconut oil for 3 to 5 minutes.
2. Stir in the peanut butter until the mixture is creamy.

3. Add the heavy cream, liquid stevia, cocoa powder, salt, and vanilla extract briskly whisking the ingredients.

4. Fill 12 silicone muffin molds halfway with the peanut butter mixture.

5. Sprinkle with peanuts.

6. Place the molds on a baking sheet and place in the freezer for at least 1 hour, or until solid.

7. Remove the chocolate-peanut cups from the molds to serve.

Cheddar Cheese Crisps

Time: 12 minutes

Serving Size: 4 servings

Prep Time: 5 minutes

Cook Time: 7 minutes

Nutritional Facts/Info:

Calories 139

Carbs 0.4 g

Fat 11.4 g

Protein 8.6 g

Ingredients:

- 1 cup cheddar cheese, grated

Directions:

1. Line two baking sheets with parchment paper.
2. Preheat the oven to 400 degrees Fahrenheit.
3. Place the cheese in 24 small circular heaps on the baking sheets.
4. Bake for 7 minutes until golden brown.
5. Set aside and remove from backing sheets after slightly cooled.

Bumblebee Muffins

Time: 30 minutes

Serving Size: 8 servings

Prep Time: 15 minutes

Cook Time: 15 minutes

Nutritional Facts/Info:

Calories 116

Carbs 10 g

Fat 10.7 g

Protein 3.6 g

Ingredients:

- ⅓ cup natural sweetener, low-calorie if preferred
- ¼ cup coconut flour
- ¼ cup almond flour
- 1 fresh lemon zest, grated
- 1 tablespoon poppy seeds
- ½ teaspoon salt
- ½ teaspoon baking powder
- 3 eggs, large
- ¼ teaspoon xanthan gum (optional)
- 2 tablespoons sour cream
- 3 tablespoons butter
- 2 tablespoons heavy whipping cream
- ½ teaspoon vanilla extract (sugar-free)

Directions:

1. Preheat the oven to 350 degrees Fahrenheit.
2. Grease a muffin tray.
3. In a mixing bowl, combine the sweetener, almond flour, coconut flour, poppy seeds, lemon zest, baking powder, cinnamon, and xanthan gum.
4. In a small bowl, beat eggs until fluffy.
5. Combine sour cream and vanilla extract in a large mixing bowl, then fold in the eggs.
6. Add dry ingredients to the wet ingredients, folding slowly until the batter is thick and creamy.
7. Spoon batter into the muffin tin until each cup is filled halfway.
8. Bake for 15 to 20 minutes or until golden brown on top.

Keto Butter Cookies

Time: 22 minutes

Serving Size: 12 servings

Prep Time: 10 minutes

Cook Time: 12 minutes

Nutritional Facts/Info:

Calories 196

Carbs 12.7 g

Fat 18.4 g

Protein 5 g

Ingredients:

- 2 cups almond flour, blanched
- 1 egg, large
- ½ cup softened butter
- 1 teaspoon vanilla extract, sugar-free
- ½ cup natural sweetener, low-calorie
- 1 teaspoon ground cinnamon

Directions:

1. Preheat the oven to 350 degrees Fahrenheit.

2. Using parchment paper, line a baking sheet.

3. In a mixing bowl, combine almond flour, egg, butter, vanilla extract, sweetener, and cinnamon. Blend well.

4. Create 1-inch balls out of the dough and space them 2 inches apart on the baking sheet.

5. Use fork tines to create a criss-cross shape on each ball.

6. Allow to bake for 12 to 15 minutes or until crispy around the edges.

7. Cool for 1 minute on a baking sheet and then cool completely on a wire rack.

Cheesy Breakfast Biscuits

Time: 40 minutes

Serving Size: 9 servings

Prep Time: 20 minutes

Cook Time: 20 minutes

Nutritional Facts/Info:

Calories 329

Carbs 7.2 g

Fat 27.1 g

Protein 16.7 g

Ingredients:

- 2 cups almond flour
- 2 ½ cups cheddar cheese, grated
- 1 tablespoon baking powder
- ¼ cup half-and-half
- 4 eggs, large

Directions:

1. Preheat the oven to 350 degrees Fahrenheit.
2. Use parchment paper to line a baking sheet.
3. In a big mixing bowl, whisk together the almond flour and baking powder.
4. Fold in the cheddar cheese.

5. In the middle of the bowl, make a shallow well. Crack eggs into the well and add half-and-half.

6. Blend in the flour mixture with a large fork or spoon until you have a moist batter.

7. Ladle 9 batter scoops onto your preheated baking dish.

8. Bake for 20 minutes or until golden.

Parmesan Zucchini Fries

Time: 15 minutes

Serving Size: 4 servings

Prep Time: 15 minutes

Cook Time: 30 minutes

Nutritional Facts/Info:

Calories 142

Carbs 10.4 g

Fat 7.2 g

Protein 11.7 g

Ingredients:

- Cooking spray
- ¾ cup Parmesan cheese, grated
- 2 eggs, large
- 1 ½ teaspoons garlic powder
- 1 tablespoon dried mixed herbs
- ½ teaspoon ground black pepper, to season
- 1 teaspoon paprika
- 2 pounds zucchinis, cut into 1/2-inch strips

Directions:

1. Preheat the oven to 425 degrees Fahrenheit.

2. Spray a baking sheet with cooking spray and line it with aluminum foil.

3. In a small bowl, whisk eggs.

4. In a separate bowl, combine Parmesan cheese, garlic powder, mixed herbs, pepper, and paprika. Stir well.

5. In batches, dip zucchini fries in egg, shake off excess, and roll in Parmesan mixture until fully covered.

6. Bake for 30 to 35 minutes, rotating once until golden and crispy.

Chapter 7: Meal Plan and Exercise Plan

Week 1
Monday

Breakfast: Bacon, Egg & Cheese Breakfast Muffins

Lunch: Easy Low-Carb Cauliflower Mac 'n Cheese

Supper: Kimchi Pork Lettuce Cups

Snack: Hot Bacon Cheese Dip

Tuesday

Breakfast: Blueberry Almond Pancakes

Lunch: Keto Beef Egg Roll Slaw

Dinner: Thai Turkey Burgers

Snack: Marinated Olive & Cheese Ring

Wednesday

Breakfast: Berry Breakfast Shake

Lunch: Cobb Salad

Dinner: BBQ Flank Steak & Cabbage Slaw

Snack: Roasted Red Pepper Tapenade

Thursday

Breakfast: Cheddar, Spinach & Mushroom Omelet

Lunch: Keto Shrimp Scampi with Broccoli Noodles

Dinner: Beef Bolognese

Snack: Cold Chicken-Cheese Kabobs

Friday

Breakfast: Personal Portobello Pizza

Lunch: Personal Portobello Pizza

Dinner: Smoky Butter Roasted Chicken

Snack: Sweet Onion Pimiento Cheese Deviled Eggs

Week 2

Monday

Breakfast: Feta Frittata

Lunch: Easy Keto Beef Tacos

Dinner: Sheet-Pan Chicken Fajita Bowls

Snack: Smoked Salmon Cheese Spread

Tuesday

Breakfast: Bacon and Asparagus Frittata

Lunch: Seafood Stuffed Avocados

Dinner: Almond-Crusted Salmon Patties

Snack: Marinated Cheese

Wednesday

Breakfast: Southwestern Omelet

Lunch: Keto Tuna Salad

Dinner: Swedish Meatballs

Snack: Feta-Stuffed Portobello Mushrooms

Thursday

Breakfast: Ham Steaks with Gruyere, Bacon & Mushrooms

Lunch: Keto Spaghetti Squash with Bacon and Blue Cheese

Dinner: Magic Keto Pizza

Snack: Sesame Chicken Dip

Friday

Breakfast: French Omelet

Lunch: Creamy Keto Cauliflower Risotto

Dinner: Citrus Saumon en Papillote

Snack: Savory Cheese Ball

Week 3
Monday

Breakfast: Homemade Sage Sausage Patties

Lunch: Cherry Chicken Lettuce Wraps

Dinner: Broiled Chicken & Artichokes

Snack: Mashed Cauliflower with Parmesan

Tuesday

Breakfast: Spinach-Mushroom Scrambled Eggs

Lunch: Easy Keto Korean Beef with Cauli Rice

Dinner: Garlic-Butter Steak

Snack: Potluck Sausage-Stuffed Mushrooms

Wednesday

Breakfast: Broccoli Quiche Cups

Lunch: Caveman Chili

Dinner: Blackened Tilapia with Zucchini Noodles

Snack: Sausage-Stuffed Jalapenos

Thursday

Breakfast: Mediterranean Broccoli & Cheese Omelet

Lunch: Taco Stuffed Avocados

Dinner: Scallops with Wilted Spinach

Snack: Bacon-Wrapped Asparagus

Friday

Breakfast: Asparagus Cream Cheese Omelet

Lunch: Buffalo Shrimp Lettuce Wraps

Dinner: Coconut Curry Cauliflower Soup

Snack: Spinach-Parm Casserole

Week 4

Monday

Breakfast: Crustless Spinach Quiche

Lunch: Keto Broccoli Salad

Dinner: Chicken and Broccoli with Dill Sauce

Snack: Grilled Jalapenos

Tuesday

Breakfast: Ham & Broccoli Frittata

Lunch: Keto Egg Salad

Dinner: Vegetable, Steak, and Eggs

Snack: Tuscan-Style Roasted Asparagus

Wednesday

Breakfast: Oven Denver Omelet

Lunch: Keto Bacon Sushi

Dinner: Mexican Cabbage Roll Soup

Snack: Ricotta-Stuffed Portobello Mushrooms

Thursday

Breakfast: Calico Scrambled Eggs

Lunch: Keto Burger Fat Bombs

Dinner: BLT Chicken Salad

Snack: Blue Cheese-Stuffed Shrimp

Friday

Breakfast: Asparagus Cream Cheese Omelet

Lunch: Sesame Beef & Asparagus Salad

Dinner: Grilled Ribeyes with Greek Relish

Snack: Jalapeno-Pecan Cheese Spread

Exercise Plan

Women over 50 often, incorrectly, living a life that is currently sedentary means that they cannot exercise once they reach 50. That assumption is, however, not true. It is never too late to begin an exercise routine that complements your healthy eating habits. Implementing regular exercise when you are over 50 can help to reverse several aches and pains that only began when you became sedentary.

Taking a look at the benefits of an exercise regime after 50, it is not difficult to see why health practitioners encourage women in this age group to get moving. Studies conducted by the Mayo Clinic staff in 2019 show that increased muscle mass and overall strength help to slow menopausal muscle degeneration effects and targets unhealthy heart health belly fat. Getting fit during this period of your life can stave off those extra pounds that often come with menopause which, in turn, lowers your chance of developing type 2 diabetes, certain cancers, and heart disease.

Having said that, not all exercises are equal. Some may need to be avoided or, at least, gradually introduced into your workout routine.

- Weight training-If you have previously lifted weights, then weight training is an option for you. Pilates and resistance bands are a great way to ease your body into weight training while still building muscle mass and increasing your strength.

- Cardiovascular and Aerobic Exercise-Also known as endurance workouts, cardio promotes heart health, burns fat, and improves circulation in the body. Swimming, walking, and organized aerobic classes are excellent cardio exercises to institute into your workout routine. If you can speak when exercising, but can feel your heart rate increasing, then you are doing cardio well.

- Stretching-Yoga, and other exercises that promote stretching are excellent for maintaining flexibility and improving joint health.

- Balance-Unfortunately, as one ages, the risk of falling increases. Exercises that promote balance such as Tai Chi help to keep your body's balance receptors in tune.

Remember that the different forms of exercise don't necessarily need to be done separately. Walking with ankle weights, for example, incorporates both cardiovascular exercises as well as weight and resistance training. As long as you have the okay from your health practitioner and are exercising responsibly, your body will respond by becoming stronger and better balanced.

As an over age 50 individual, you should be aiming for 150 minutes of moderate exercise each week or, if you are transitioning from a previous exercise routine, 75 minutes of vigorous activity each week. This can be broken down into 30 minutes five times a week for moderate exercise, or 15 minutes of vigorous activity five times a week. Doctors recommend that 10 minutes of strength training should be done at least twice a week by individuals over age 50. For those who have limited mobility, or who want to improve their balance, an additional 15 minutes, three days each week should be set aside to incorporate balancing exercises.

Strength Training for Over

Strength training does not require extensive gym equipment, although working out at your local gym does give you access to this machinery and encourages socialization. If you want to incorporate strength training at home, however, a simple resistance band and bodyweight movements, like squats and push-ups, will also yield good results.

Plank Pose-Planking can help correct posture, strengthen and tone your abdominal muscles, and improve balance. For over 50s, planking in the push-up position alleviates discomfort on the forearms and elbows. If you have experience planking or feel you need more of a challenge, a traditional plank pose on your forearms can be performed. Remember to keep your core engaged and your back straight when planking.

Hold your plank pose until 'fail,' which means that you absolutely cannot stay up any longer.

Chair Squats-Squatting promotes balance and builds the gluteal and thigh muscles. There are numerous variations of the squat that can be incorporated into your exercise routine to work different muscle groups.

Place a chair under your rear, keep your back straight, and put your arms straight out in front of your chest, lower your body by bending your legs until your behind is just above the chair. Repeat this motion for 12 counts and repeat three times throughout your workout.

Chest Fly-This exercise, while traditionally done with weights in the gym, does not require the use of weights. Filled water bottles, a resistance band, or cans of food will work equally as well. Instead of lying on a bench, as you would at the gym, you can lie on the floor. Chest flies work the pectoral muscles and build arm and upper back strength.

Lie on your back, bend your knees and make sure your feet are flat on the ground. Slide your arms out straight so that your body forms a T, bending your elbows to 90 degrees. Slowly lift your weighted arms one at a time until they are at a 90-degree angle in the air. In a controlled motion, return your arm to its starting position and lift your other arm, repeating the exercise. Do 12 repetitions on each arm and repeat three times throughout your workout.

Yoga For Over 50s

Yoga is the most popular form of exercise for women over 50 in the United States. Over 40% of all over 50's in the US either practice yoga at their local gym, club, or at home (Wei, 2016). There are numerous forms of yoga, so be sure to do your homework before instituting it into your workout routine. This ensures you are not signing up for a particularly rigorous form of this exercise. If you have not practiced yoga before, and wish to try incorporating it into your home workout, you can begin with yoga that utilizes a chair; this is less strenuous than other forms of yoga.

Downward Facing Dog

Place your chair with the seating area against a wall and the backrest facing you. Stand approximately two feet from the front edge of your chair and crouch down. Slowly lift your rear towards the ceiling, keeping your feet firmly placed in their starting position. Slowly raise your body upwards, arms above your head, stretching at your highest point. Hold for 30 seconds before slowly bending forward from your hips, until your hands are resting on the chair seating. Keeping your knees bent, and your hands on the chair seat, slowly walk your legs back until you create arms form a diagonal line to your torso and hips. For advanced stretchers, your hands should not lift off the floor as your rear rises into the air, and no chair is required.

To come out of your pose, bend your knees and slowly walk your feet forward, towards the chair. Once you are approximately a foot from the chair, lift your torso from your hips until you are in an upright standing position.

Seated Forward Bend

With the backrest of your chair pushed against a wall, sit with your legs stretched straight out in front of you. Lift your arms straight above your head, inhaling, before slowly bending forward towards your toes. Hold your pose for 30 seconds when the stretch feels uncomfortable but bearable. Once you can comfortably reach your toes and hold the pose, you can graduate to sitting on the floor and slowly working your way down to your toes. Make sure your legs remain straight and don't arch your back.

Low Plank Pose

Also known as the yoga half push up, the low plank pose is a powerful exercise that activates a host of muscles in the body. The low plank works by strengthening and stretching your arms, torso, and legs.

Beginning in a neutral stance, or from downward dog, and facing the seating area of your chair, stretch your arms straight above your head. Bend forward from your hips until your palms are in the center of the chair's seating area. Inhale deeply, walking your feet backward until your spine, and legs are straight. Slowly lower your arms forwards, and downwards towards the chair until you are in a push-up position. Hold this position for six breath counts. Return to your starting position by straightening your arms until they are 90 degrees to the chair. Slowly lift your torso from the hips until you are in a standing position.

Cardio for Over 50s

After the age of 50, cardiovascular and aerobics exercises should be low impact and gentle on your joints. If at all possible, swimming twice a week is an amazing, low-impact workout that activates and strengthens all of your muscles while improving lung function and heart health. Most local health clubs and gyms offer fun, muscle building, fat burning water aerobics classes that are specifically designed to reduce pressure on your joints.

If swimming isn't your cup of tea, try brisk walking or spending time on the treadmill at your local gym. Outdoor walking is especially useful in building endurance and activating different muscle groups as the terrain changes. According to a study conducted by Harvard Medical School in 2010, spending time outdoors has also been shown to greatly improve a person's mood and encourages dopamine responses in the brain.

1 Week Workout Schedule

Monday

- Start your day with 10 minutes of yoga, making sure not to rush through your poses.
- Before breakfast 30-minute mini-aerobic workout.

Tuesday

- Start your day with a 10-minute deep stretch to ease aching muscles.
- Midday resistance or weighted exercise for 30 minutes. Make sure to fuel your body afterward with a wholesome lunch.

Wednesday

Rest day

Thursday

- Stretch and start your day with 10 minutes of yoga.
- Late afternoon fast/slow walking session for 30 minutes.

Friday

- 10 minutes of home aerobic workout to help you feel energized all day.
- 30 minutes of resistance or weight exercise before lunch. Wind down with a wholesome meal.

Saturday

- Start your day with a 10-minute stretch to ease your muscles.
- Spend 30 minutes in the pool or 30 minutes outdoors, using a fast/slow pace.

Sunday

Rest day. However, I encourage you to practice 10 minutes of yoga first thing in the morning so that you feel refreshed for the remainder of the day.

Conclusion

Intermittent fasting has become a worldwide health trend with a difference. IF encourages a person to eat according to their natural circadian rhythms. Studies have shown that these eating cycles between fasting and eating increase the overall health of a person (Welto, 2020). The added benefit of weight loss and the prevention of age-specific diseases makes intermittent fasting an option that over 50s should be seriously considering.

IF, when combined with a scientifically proven healthy eating plan, produces dramatically positive health results. IF focuses more on the time and time between meals and not as much on the specific foods you put in your body. you 'when' you should be eating, making it easier, most cost-effective, and more manageable to integrate into your busy schedule.

Throughout human evolution, fasting has been used to reset a person's metabolic clock or, simply, to refuel after being unable to locate food for extended periods. Because the process of intermittent fasting stems from evolution, science has shown that the human body can, and will, survive without food for an extended period when fueled correctly outside the eating windows.

While the most common fasting regime involves fasting for 16 hours, other forms of fasting can be instituted into your specific lifestyle. For most though, the 16/8 method works as it can be easily incorporated into a person's modern-day lifestyle. When you choose to fast, several biological processes occur in your body. These biological responses include an increase in HGH, the fat-burning hormone, insulin stabilization, and cellular repair. Beyond these positive biological responses, intermittent fasting is an incredible weight loss tool and has been shown to increase your metabolic rate by between 3.6% and 14% (Duan, et al, 2016).

Combining intermittent fasting with a ketogenic diet and an exercise regime creates a powerhouse of healthy behaviors that benefit both your mind and body. Following a keto diet after the age of 50 encourages joint health, weight loss, and improved hormone and cholesterol levels. Eating a great balance of keto-approved vegetables, meats, and unprocessed carbs makes the ketogenic diet one that is easy to follow.

It is important to remember though that neither keto nor IF are dieting fads. Rather, they are lifestyle changes that encourage overall health and wellness. There are no 3-hour workouts, crash diets, or starvation tactics at play. These two proven methods are science-backed and adequately researched by nutritionists and general health practitioners the world over. With proper instruction and adherence to the advice in this book, any side effects to implementing your new diet should be minimized, aside from the positive effect of weight loss, of course.

Science-backed keto and intermittent fasting are often used separately, with many people wondering if the two should be combined. The answer, of course, is yes! These two eating methods go back to the dawn of humanity, before refined foods and take-aways threatened our health. With IF's aim to eat within your prescribed calorie intake and keto replenishing your body with the vitamins, minerals, and fats that it needs to function at its prime, the combination of the two eating regimes provides a unique set of benefits that other dietary fads cannot.

Shown to control blood sugar levels, reduce inflammation, and improve cognitive brain function as well as encouraging regeneration on a cellular level, intermittent fasting is the go-to for nutritionists and doctors around the world (Little, 2020). Keto on the other hand has been used for centuries to improve the brain function of those suffering from neurological diseases such as Epilepsy and Alzheimers. Added to this, the ketogenic diet lowers LDL cholesterol, promotes good heart health, and encourages a healthy circulatory system (Duan, et al, 2016).

When these two healthy lifestyles are combined, studies have shown that IF assists the body into ketosis (Duan, et al, 2016), a state of fat burning quicker because insulin and glycogen reserves are diminished and the body is forced to burn fat for fuel. This, of course, leads to more fat being eliminated from the body, but, because keto replenishes your body with healthy foods, muscle mass is not affected. Additional studies have shown that, when keto and intermittent fasting are combined, hunger is significantly reduced (van de Walle, 2018). Because the ketogenic diet reduces hunger and promotes feelings of fullness, the chances of breaking one's fast before the required time becomes less probable.

For you to remain on track with your intermittent fasting lifestyle, you should begin your journey by first introducing a ketogenic lifestyle. This will help you to become accustomed to the richness of the food and also get you into the routine of making healthy food choices for yourself and your family. Once you are used to your new way of eating, you can begin to ease yourself into IF. For most people, the 16/8 fasting protocol works well because the majority of your fasting hours fall in line with your sleep cycle. Your choice of fasting plan, however, is entirely up to you. When instituting keto, IF, and exercise into your life, you can begin to reverse the effects of a sedentary lifestyle. Many people believe that if they have lived a life that was low activity or sedentary, they cannot begin an exercise plan when they reach their 50s. This is not true! Exercise, along with a healthy eating lifestyle offers huge rewards and benefits. Remaining active and incorporating strength or weight training, as well as stretching and balance exercises into your life, not only assists in weight loss but with other aspects of your overall health. Consistent exercise reduces your risk of heart disease, high blood pressure, diabetes, and stroke, while studies have shown that it also keeps your mind mentally alert. Inflammatory and degenerative diseases are shown to significantly slow with just 30 minutes of moderate exercise a day (Welto, 2020). Besides these amazing health benefits, exercise encourages time outdoors and in social settings which is excellent for your mental health.

If you are still unsure as to whether intermittent fasting combined with a ketogenic diet is for you, consider this: What do you have to lose by trying? In as little as a month, you stand to lose weight, feel healthier, fitter, and more satisfied with your body's strength level and overall health. Your age does not need to be the end of your health journey. It may be the beginning.

References

Abstract. (2005). *Breast Cancer Research and Treatment, 94* (Suppl 1), S1–S301. https://doi.org/10.1007/s10549-005-1234-6

Allrecipes | Food, friends, and recipe inspiration. (2019). https://www.allrecipes.com/

Benefits of intermittent fasting for women over 50. (2019, May 31). Plate. https://www.primewomenplate.com/benefits-of-intermittent-fasting-for-women-over-50

Best Exercises for Women Over 50. (2019, June 14). Gateway Region YMCA. https://gwrymca.org/blog/best-exercises-women-over-50

Bird, P. J. (2002, September 23). *Why does fat deposit on the hips and thighs of women and around the stomachs of men?* Scientific American. https://www.scientificamerican.com/article/why-does-fat-deposit-on-t/#:~:text=Hormones%20drive%20the%20deposition%20of

Butler, N. (2019, April 5). *Intermittent fasting for weight loss: 5 tips to start.* Medical News Today. https://www.medicalnewstoday.com/articles/324882#make-the-calories-count

Carter, A. (2019, May 31). *Does insulin make you gain weight? Causes and management.* Medical News Today. https://www.medicalnewstoday.com/articles/325328#:~:text=Insulin%20is%20a%20hormone%20that

Compton, G. (2018, January 21). *Best exercise routines for women over 50.* Skinny Ms. https://skinnyms.com/best-exercise-routines-for-women-over-50-10/

Divers, J. (2020, August 9). *National diabetes statistics report, 2020.* Centers for Disease Control and Prevention. https://www.cdc.gov/diabetes/data/statistics-report/index.html?CDC_AA_refVal=https%3A%2F%2Fwww.cdc.gov%2Fdiabetes%2Fdata%2Fstatistics%2Fstatistics-report.html

Duan, J., Rubini, A., Volek, J. S., & Grimaldi, K. A. (2013). Beyond weight loss: a review of the therapeutic uses of very-low-carbohydrate (ketogenic) diets. *European Journal of Clinical Nutrition, 67(8),* 789–796. https://doi.org/10.1038/ejcn.2013.116

Gleeson, J. (2020, April 20). *Intermittent fasting: Is it right for you?* Michigan Health. https://healthblog.uofmhealth.org/wellness-prevention/intermittent-fasting-it-right-for-you#:~:text=Besides%20weight%20loss%2C%20are%2 othere

Gunnars, K. (2020, January 2). *6 Popular Ways to Do Intermittent Fasting.* Healthline. http://www.healthline.com/nutrition/6-ways-to-do-intermittent-fasting#TOC_TITLE_HDR_7

Harvard Medical School. (2010, July 1). *Spending time outdoors is good for you, from the Harvard Health letter.* Harvard Health Publishing.

https://www.health.harvard.edu/press_releases/spending-time-outdoors-is-good-for-you

Huizen, J. (February 1, 2021). *Could intermittent fasting reduce breast cancer risk in obesity?* Medical News Today. https://www.medicalnewstoday.com/articles/could-intermittent-fasting-reduce-breast-cancer-risk-in-obesity

Little, J. (n.d.). *Scientists discover new benefit for low-carb breakfast.* Inverse. https://www.inverse.com/article/56303-reversed-circadian-rhythm-type-2-diabetes-blood-sugar-breakfast

Lots of Yoga. (n.d.). *Yoga Over 50 - 14 Yoga Poses That You Can Do At Any Age.* Lots of Yoga. https://lotsofyoga.com/blogs/yoga-tips/yoga-over-50-best-yoga-poses

Migala, J. (2019, January 29). *Intermittent fasting on keto: How it works, benefits, risks, more.* Everyday Health. https://www.everydayhealth.com/ketogenic-diet/intermittent-fasting-keto-how-it-works-benefits-risks-more/

Nazario, B. (2020, August 19). *Slideshow: Over 50? These problems can sneak up on you.* Compass by WebMD. https://www.webmd.com/healthy-aging/ss/slideshow-health-problems-after-50

Peters, J. (2020, December 7). *21 keto-friendly lunch recipes made for low-carb lovers.* Delish. https://www.delish.com/cooking/nutrition/g28229401/keto-lunch-ideas/?slide=4

Taste of Home. (2019). https://www.tasteofhome.com/

Van De Walle, G. (2018). *The best macronutrient ratio for weight loss.* Healthline. https://www.healthline.com/nutrition/best-macronutrient-ratio

Printed in Great Britain
by Amazon